I0435824

*"Everybody needs beauty as well as bread,
places to play in and pray in, where nature
may heal and give strength to body and soul."*

—John Muir

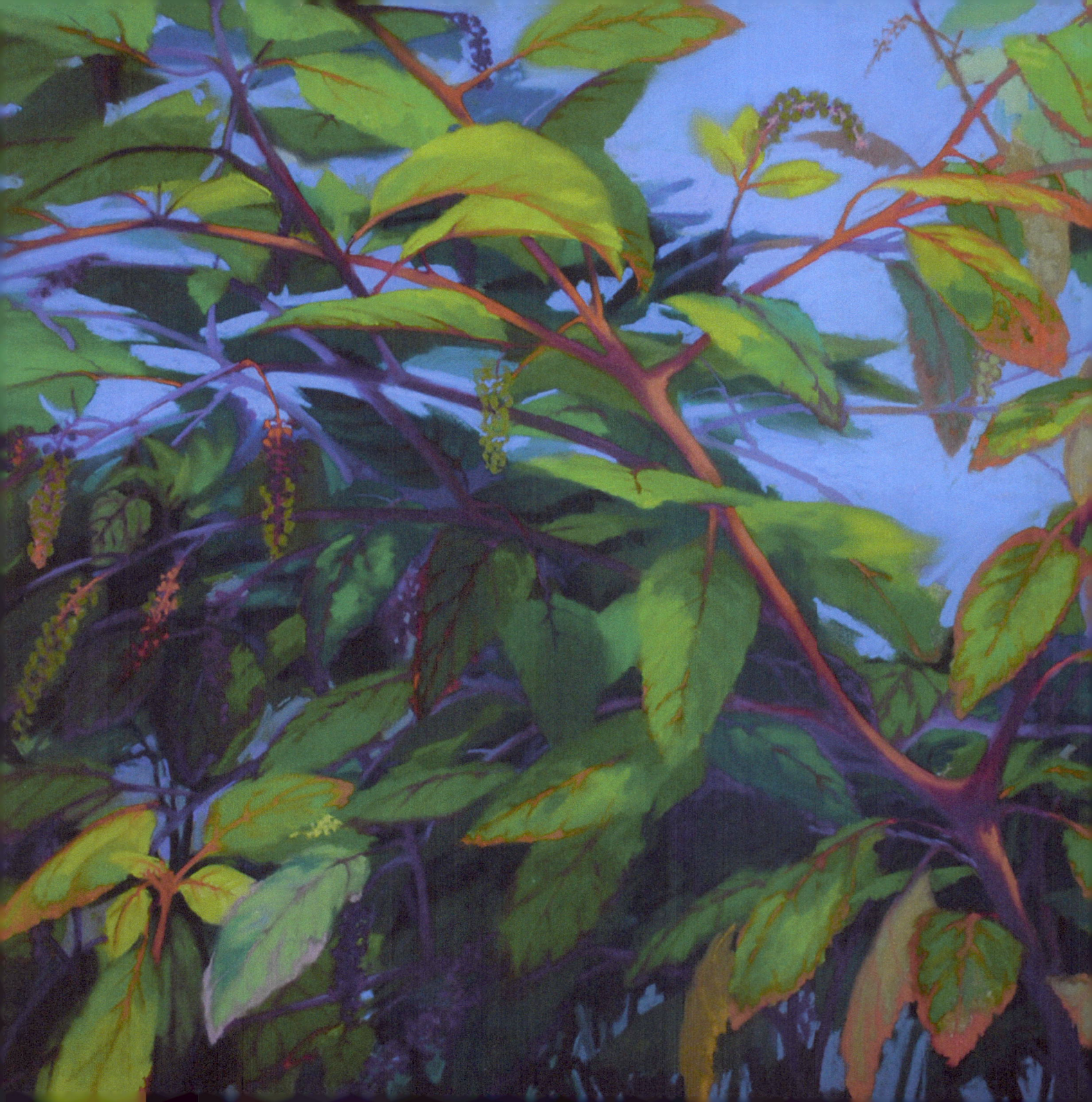

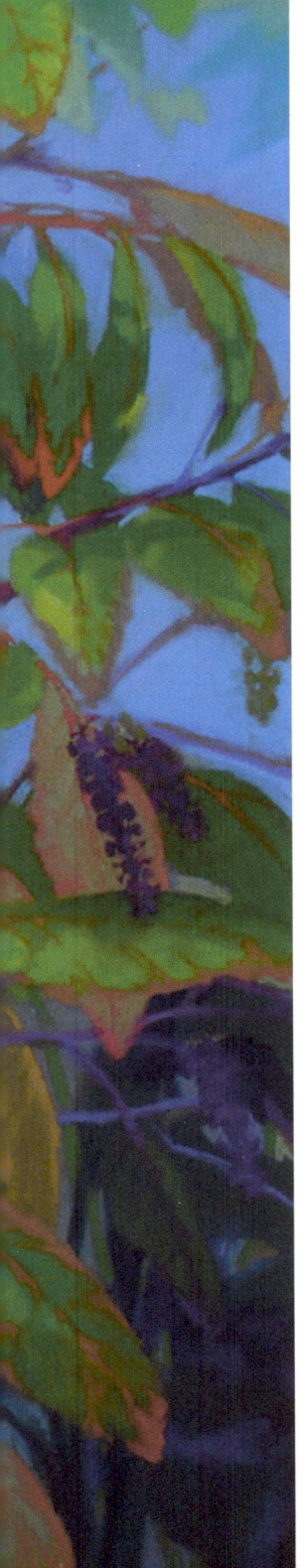

PASTEL PAINTING IS TRANSCENDENTAL

A Plein Air Diary

by Alexia Scott, MFA

Left Image: *Independence,* **Pastel on Wallis white sanded paper, 40 in. x 50 in. by Alexia Scott, July 2009**

This common Virginia weed was a very independent weed in my garden. Every year it grew up from the roots which were embedded with the roots of a lilac bush. One beautiful morning, the light inspired me to paint the Pokeweed rather than cut it out. The painting was started outside in the garden and finished in my studio at the Torpedo Factory Art Center in Alexandria, VA. Visitors made comments about a Poke Salad Festival in Louisiana. I knew the plant was poisonous and thought I should look for more information. I found that colonial Americans made ink from the berries and wrote *The Declaration of Independence* with this berry ink.

Green Pigment Publications

Artwork & Photography: Alexia Scott
Project Editor: Linda Scott
Marketing Director: Alexandra Koury
Book Design: Marinda Scott

Right Image: *Clearing Storm,* Pastel, 24 in. x 24. in.
by Alexia Scott, June 2009

First Edition
Copyright ©2014 Alexia Scott. All rights reserved. ISBN 978-0-9915547-0-6

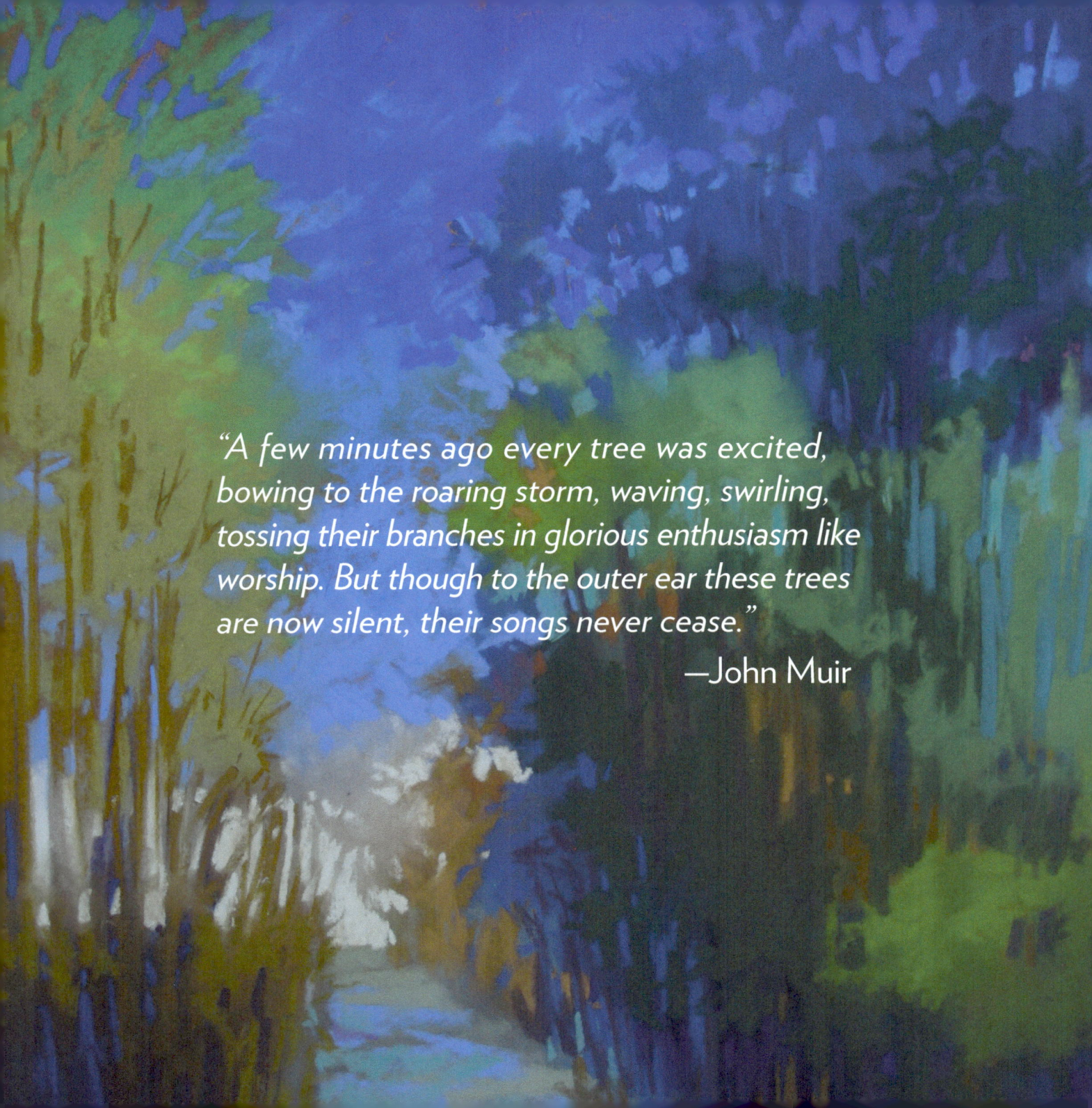

"A few minutes ago every tree was excited, bowing to the roaring storm, waving, swirling, tossing their branches in glorious enthusiasm like worship. But though to the outer ear these trees are now silent, their songs never cease."

—John Muir

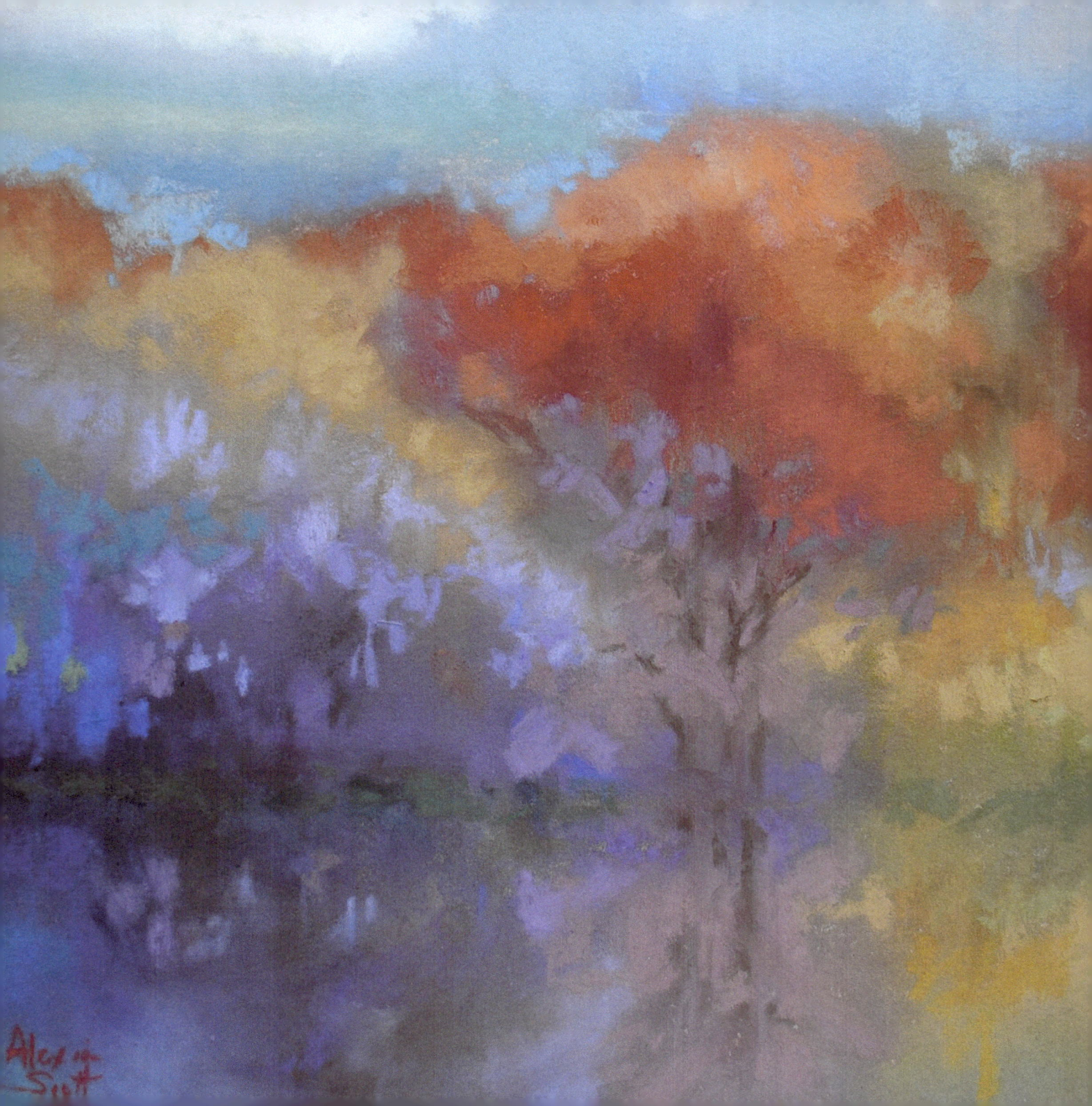

Table of Contents

Left Image: *Across the Potomac,* Pastel, 12 in. x 12 in.
by Alexia Scott, October 2010
Painted from my studio window at the Torpedo Factory Art Center. When you cannot be outside, you can work from a window.

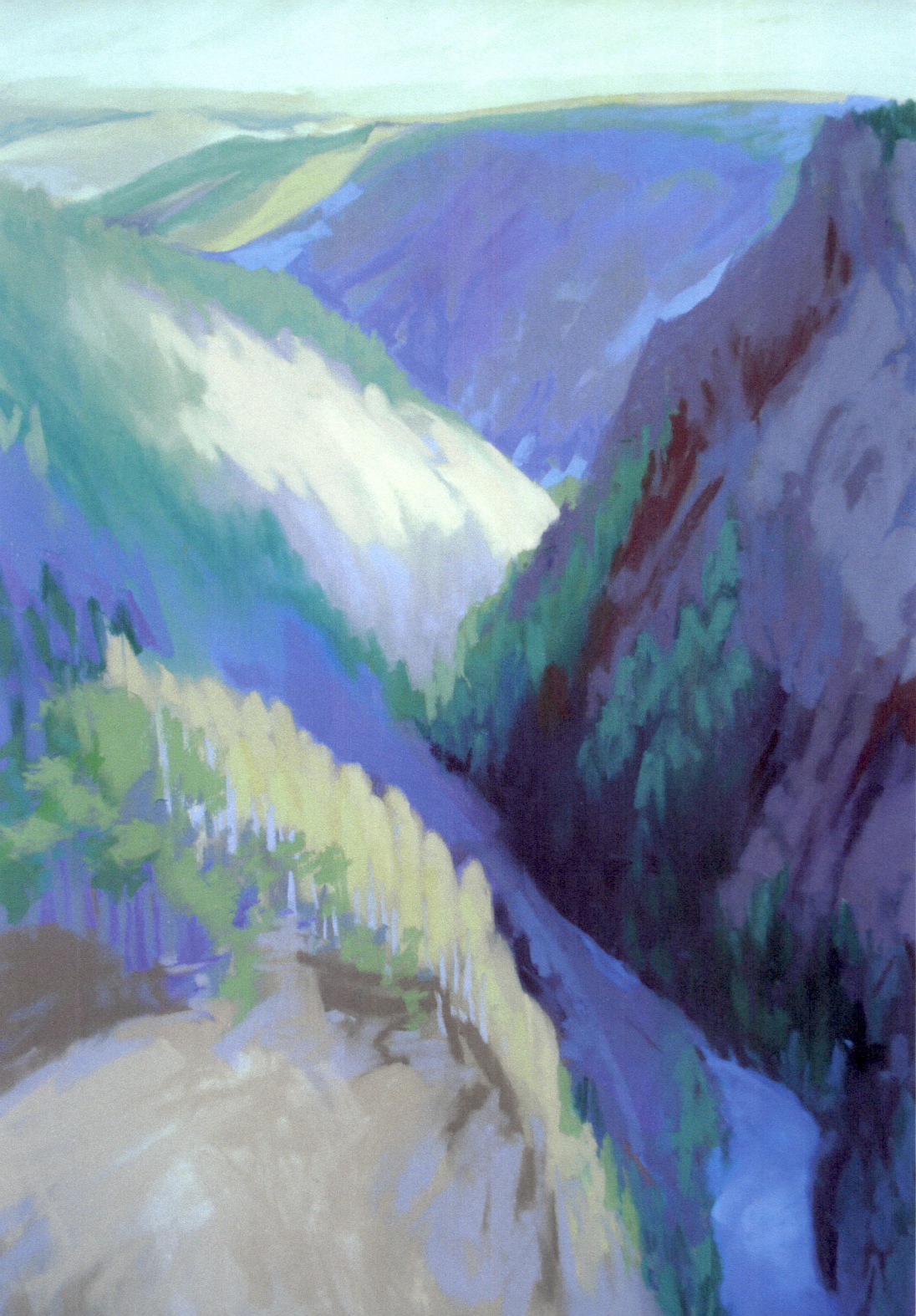

This book is dedicated to Thomas W. Scott, M.D.,
who has put up with my pastel dust for many years, and
shared his medical knowledge which inspired this book.

Left Image: *Yellowstone Canyon*, Pastel on Wallis sanded white paper, 20 in. x 30 in.
by Alexia Scott, August 2009
I painted this facing north at Artist Point along the canyon rim.

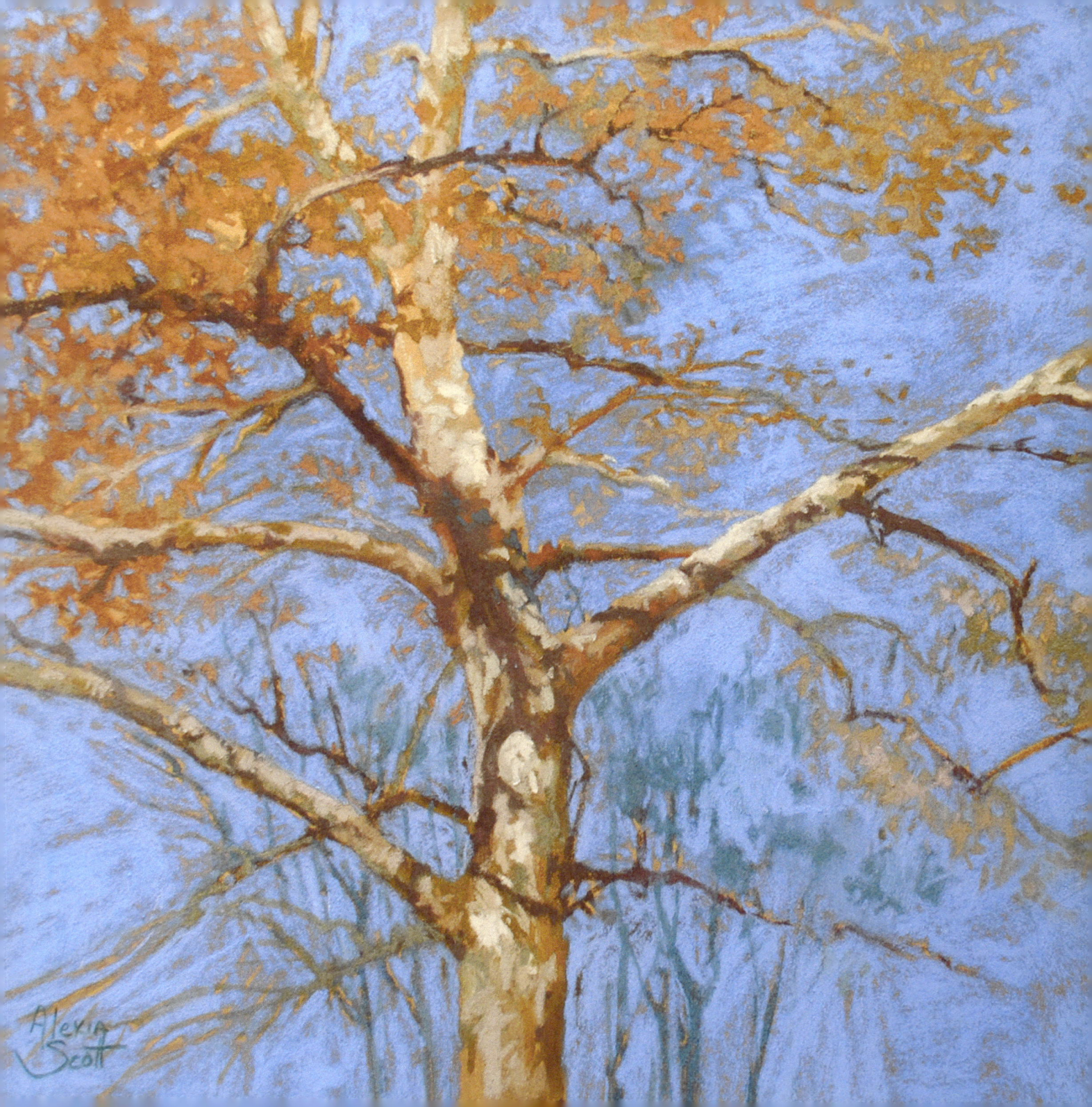

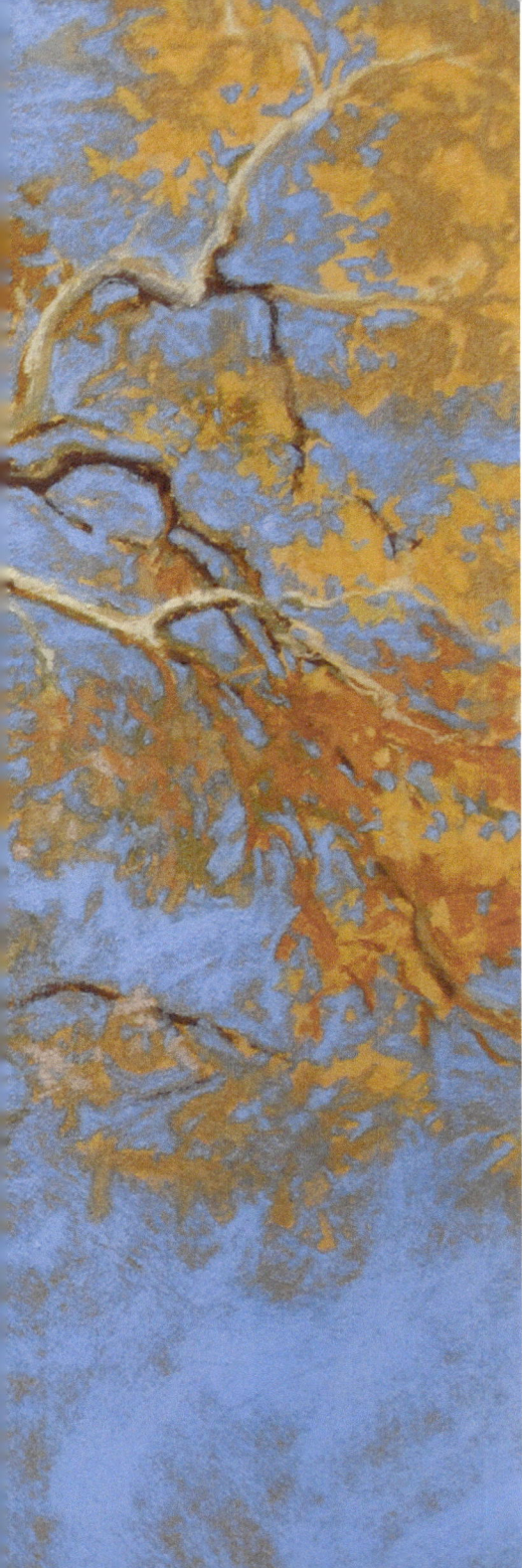

Art as Therapy

This book is not about words but soft marks of pure pigment color. It is about contemplation of nature and color. Over the course of a lifetime, we develop a vocabulary for a visual language. A transcendental basis of visual knowledge that is independent of our conscious experiences. This book explores a universal language of color and nature and how this exploration can improve our mental well-being.

On September 11, 2001, across the river from the Pentagon at Georgetown University, my students felt the ground shake as the plane hit the Pentagon's west side. The next day, I walked into a full classroom of silent students. Before leaving home, I cut branches from my Chinese chestnut tree encrusted with nut pods. I brought the outside into the classroom knowing that drawing from nature might help and drawing outside was possibly dangerous. For two hours, we drew each stem and leaf following

Left Image: *Sycamore with Golden Leaves,* **Pastel, 18 in. x 20 in. by Alexia Scott, Pastel on LaCarte Pastel Card, December 2013**
An early morning winter walk provided this blue sky and gold leaves for me to paint. Winter has some striking colors and working from a window still renews the mind and spirit.

the contour of the edges and spines of the nut pods. There was no talking and no music; only nature, eyes, hands, and a pen. At the end of the class, every student, and myself realized that for two hours our right brain had completely blocked our anxiety. Nothing had changed, but we had changed our state of mind from anxious to calm...at least for a short time. The focus necessary to carefully draw the branch and leaves blocked out all other thoughts. This was not a class of art majors. The students were from many cultures, male and female, crew team members, basketball players, pre-med students, and political science majors, and they all felt the same way...a brief sense of relief.

All art teachers understand the healing benefits of making art and how it helps to understand the individual student through analysis of their artwork. When a student begins to draw in an obviously new heavy-handed method, you can be fairly certain life has become strenuous. When asked, they will generally tell you the problem but they need to be noticed. I once opened a student's portfolio to see all of their work cut in to small 3-inch triangles. This spoke volumes. I find it particularly distressing that so many school systems have eliminated art from their curriculum. From the beginning, one of our first acts is to make pictures. Our world surrounds us with visual communication; from everything we buy through advertising to how the front page of the newspaper is designed to catch our attention. Nothing is accidental.

One day a young man walked into my studio at the Torpedo Factory Art Center and asked me if any artist at the art center created "socially relevant art". I thought for a moment and responded that through my knowledge of color and form, I tried to created imagery of nature that made the viewer respond in a calm and meditative way. He said he was an anarchist. Working in an art center is a unique way to absorb daily feedback on ones own work and how the viewer relates to the work.

This is how I learned what I will share with you. How do we use this creative process to improve our mind, calm our nerves, and brighten our day?

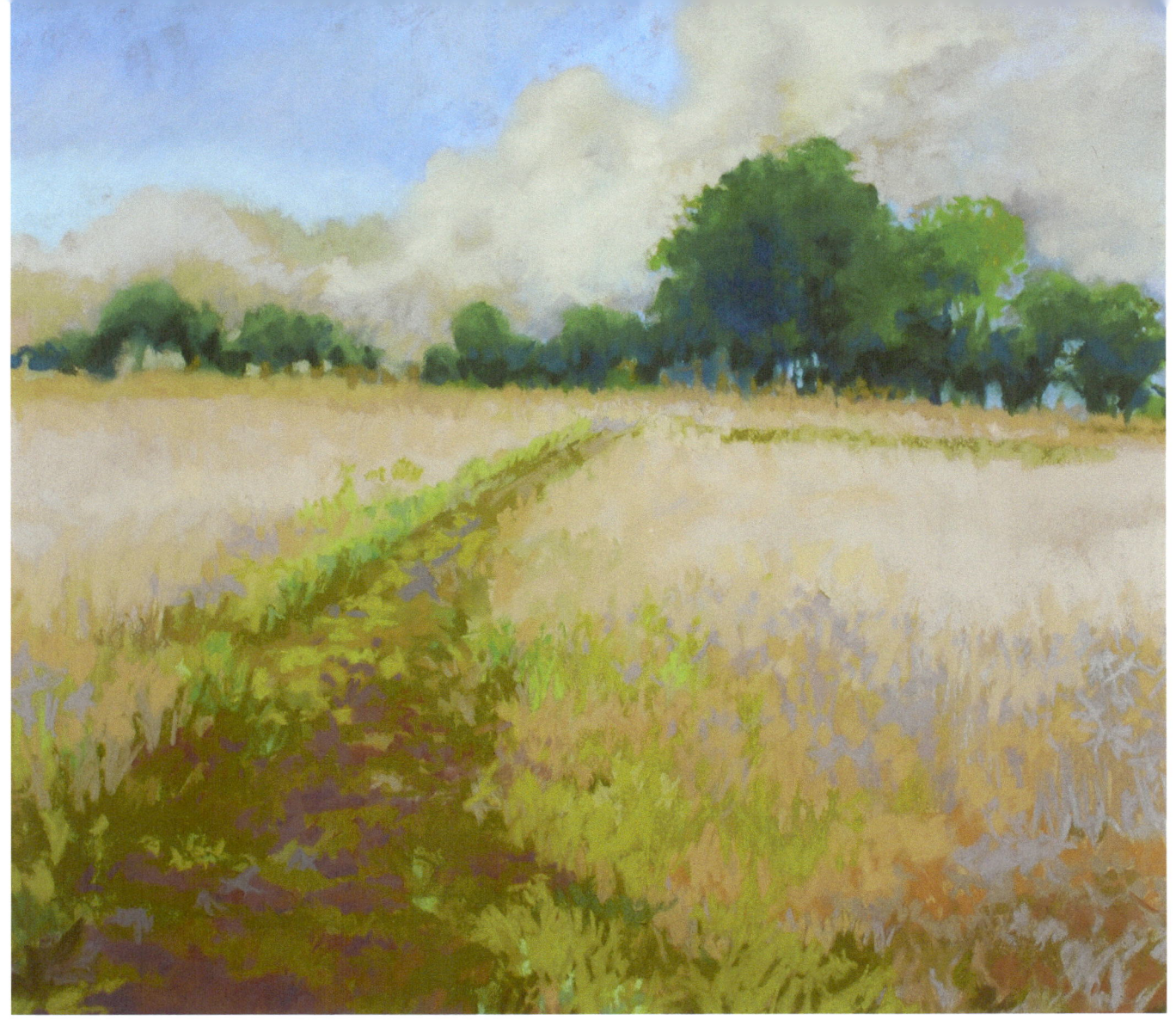

Favorite Path, Pastel on La Carte Pastel Card, 19 in. x 20 in.
by Alexia Scott, July 2013

Big Meadows in Shenandoah National Park, VA, is a location I visit several times during the year. The meadow is a beautiful place with native flowers and wildlife. It is a calm location on the mountaintop and begs to be painted again and again at every season.

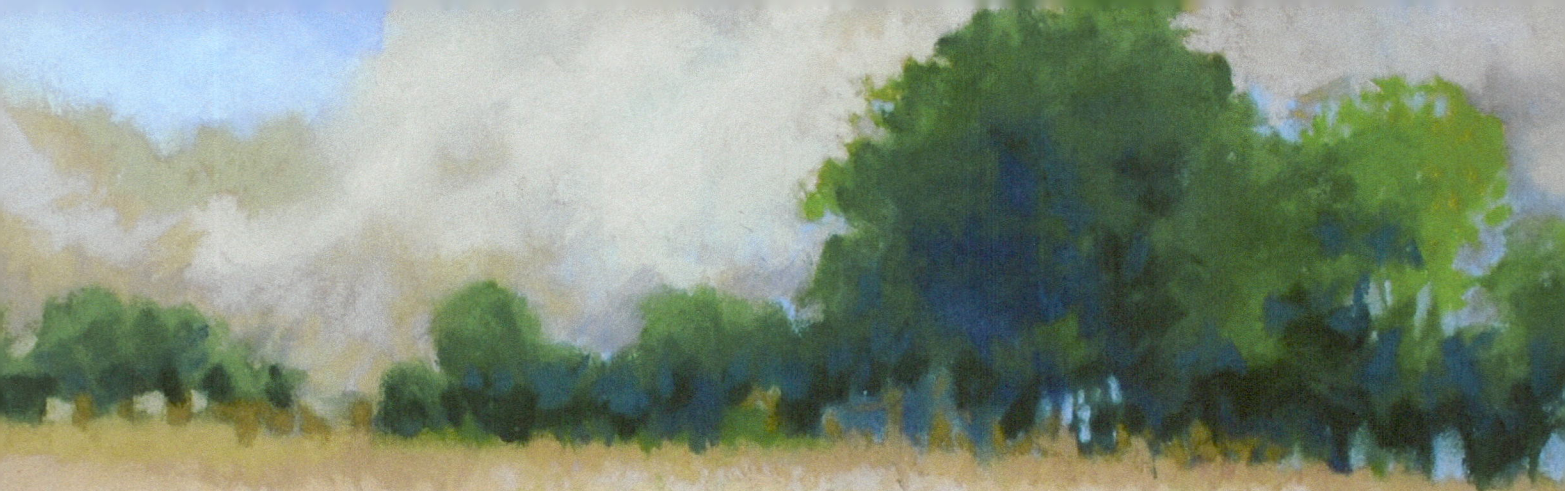

Why Pastel Pigments

The transcendental nature of pastel painting suggests that there is a common connection between us and these pigments, colors, and image-making sticks that transforms our studies. Some of our first creative achievements as mankind were pastel paintings. Found in the caves of Chauvet and Lascaux in modern day France, these paintings document our need to express ourselves visually and in color. The pastel paintings in the Chauvet caves date from 32,000 – 30,000 BP. Here we find hundreds of animal paintings created using pigments of native minerals and charred wood. We also find handprints, the artist's signature, in red ochre earth. Red ochre is a pigment we still use today.

Our greatest gift has been this gift of creativity and the desire to communicate with others. These early image galleries of Paleolithic man also transcend language. It is fortunate for us that early man did not have a written language. Chances are we never would have been able to interpret it. Their visual language speaks to us clearly through all the years between us. Before we built cities, we made pastel paintings.

This visual vocabulary of color, form, pigments, and nature is in our DNA and I believe we are happiest allowing time in our lives to explore nature and to express ourselves. The regular practice of pastel painting can provide new mental exercises, increase your observation skills, and draw out your creativity. You will see the places you visit as you have never seen them before.

Color is contextual. It surrounds us and we respond to it emotionally, but our response varies depending on where we are and what we are doing. Recently, I walked into a local restaurant that had just redecorated with blue-violet neon lights around the top of the four walls. Blue lighting is unappetizing. Rarely do you see blue plates. Yet the same color on a pastel painting of an ocean coast makes it beautiful and inviting. It is best not to paint your powder room yellow because everyone looking in the mirror will look slightly ill, yet it is beautiful in a field of sunlit sunflowers. The images you hang on your office wall or use to decorate your home also have an effect on you and your visitors. Visual décor is a subliminal greeting that suggests to your guests how you want to relate to others.

When you introduce color into your painting, you will need to make a thousand choices. Each choice is neither right nor wrong but relates to the context of each pastel mark in your painting. With pastel pigments you are limited to what you have at hand. With oil, acrylic, and watercolor paints, you can mix just what you need, but finding and choosing the pastel colors you want to use can make for some exciting hunting. Our creativity is our legacy as humans and we should practice it for our own well-being.

Pastel painting is an essay of color instead of words, providing a mental escape and lasting thoughts. As you work with your pastel colors, absorbing and reading the landscape, you are making mental notes as well as your marks on the paper. When you visit your paintings again, you will enjoy the experience once more.

Pastel Painting En Plein Air

We belong to the outdoors, whether at the seaside or in the meadow. We feel our best there. We need warm sun, morning light, and many colors for our mental health. En Plein Air is the French phrase for painting in the open air. The French Impressionists were able to paint outside due to an important invention—the paint tube. I paint outside with pastels because they are always ready to carry, quick to set up, and I can work on my lap to paint the view. I travel with pastels because they do not require extra equipment and they are not flammable, unlike paint tubes. My primary medium is oil paint, but creating my nature studies with pastels has taken on a life of its own. Choosing colors, rather than mixing colors, adds a new color consciousness to your work. You begin to experiment in new ways and the soft pastel pigments are touchable and forgiving.

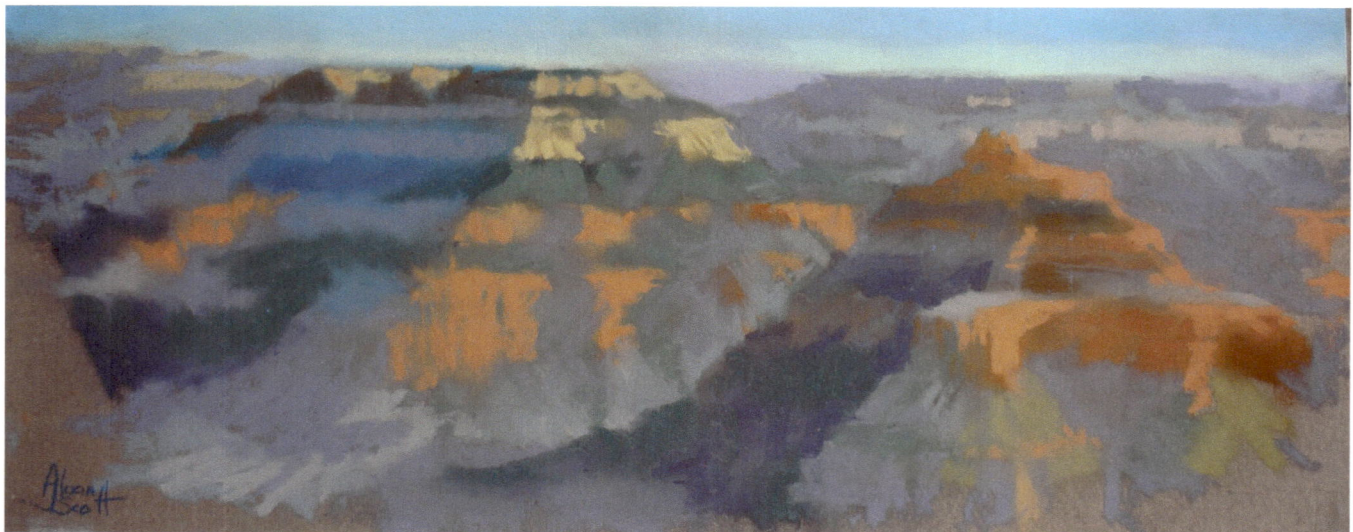

The Grand Canyon, **Pastel on Wallis sanded paper Belgian mist, 10.5 in. x 23 in. by Alexia Scott, April 2011.**

With pastels as your medium, you will never have just what you need out in the field. You are forced to experiment with color in a new way. Pastel pigments allow you to doodle your way through a study—no pressure, just observations. The canyon is the most challenging place to make a pastel. With so many layers of rock and distant planes, keeping your place is difficult. El Tovar lodge, where this pastel was done, is one of the oldest in the park, dating back to the early 1900's. It was placed in a beautiful location for painters.

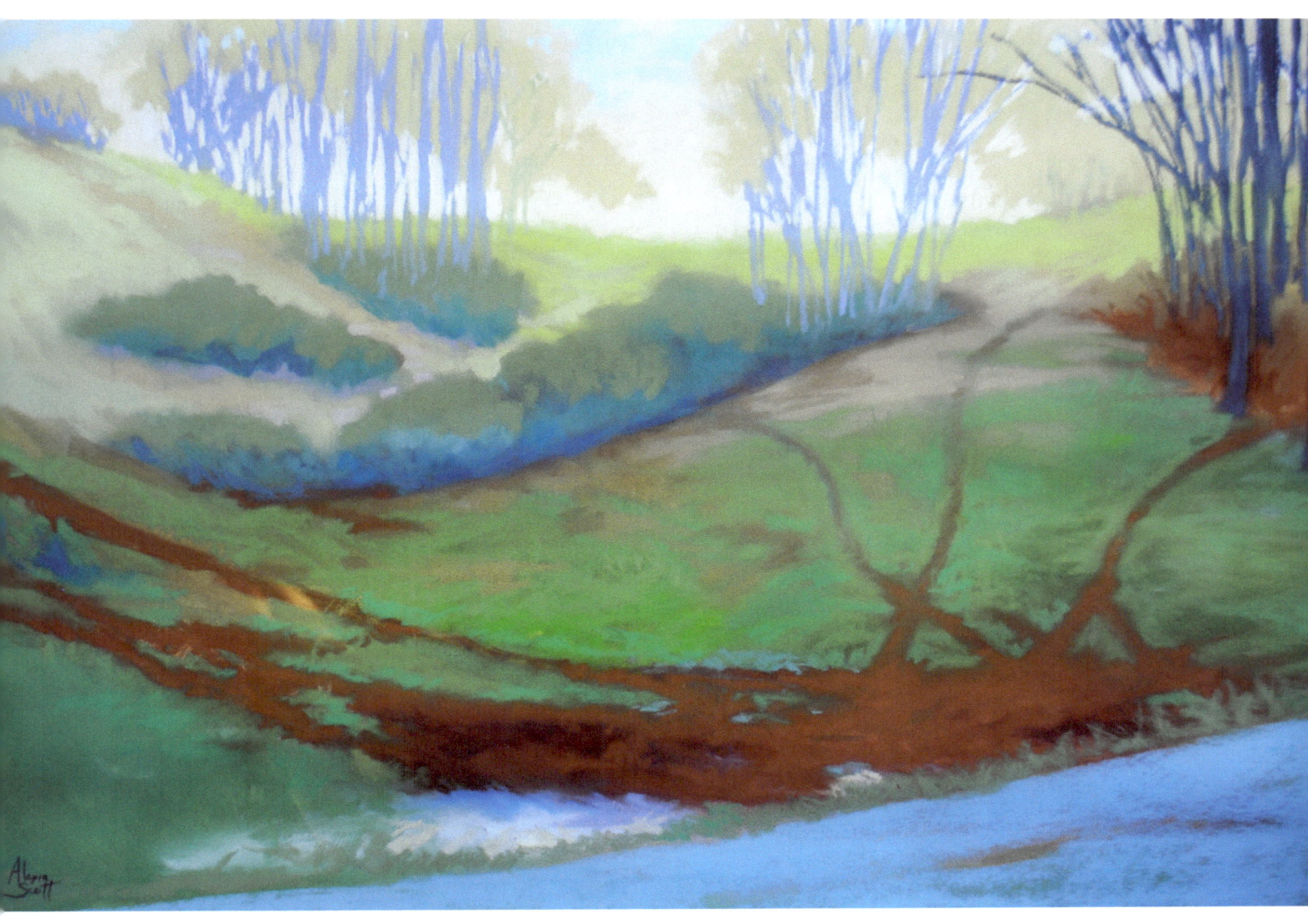

Upperville Path, Pastel on Wallis sanded paper, 20 in. x 30 in.
by Alexia Scott, April 2011

Let's Get Started with Supplies

Supplies can be as minimal as a 9 in. x 10 in. box of Half Sticks and a small pad of pastel papers, or as expansive as hundreds of different colors of pastels. I have suggested some materials to help you begin painting quickly and supplies that are easy to carry out in the field. You will find that you will get just as much enjoyment from opening the new box of pastels as you did when you were a child. Some things about us never change, they just lay dormant. Wolf Kahn, a pastel painter and teacher, once commented in class that each time he bought a new pastel color he began to see the color everywhere in the landscape.

Pastels: Hard, medium, and soft pastels can all mix (no oil pastels).
Fiber-Castell Goldfaber Soft Pastel: Set of 72 Half Sticks, pictured right, is a student grade set but has a wonderful selection of colors in a small box. Half Sticks are used up quickly but can be replaced with a similar open stock color in another brand, such as Nupastels.

Prismacolor Nupastel 96: This is the set I start my students with. These are widely used by pastel artists and designers at all levels. They are available open stock, so you can replace individual sticks. This set is larger and more expensive, but is still easy to carry and store. Both sets are good quality pastel sticks. The square sticks have the advantage of making marks with the edge and corner for finer lines. The square sticks also don't roll off your drawing board. They all work fine together and you can keep adding colors.

Right Image: I pulled all of this out of a bag I keep in my car. This is all you need to start: pastels, clips, board, paper, hand towel, water, and bug spray. A phone is helpful if you fall into a hole or are stalked by an angry crow. When you sit quietly, you will see a great deal of wildlife. Often I sit on a log and work on my lap, but you can also carry a folding field chair and a plein air-type easel, which I do when I have more time.

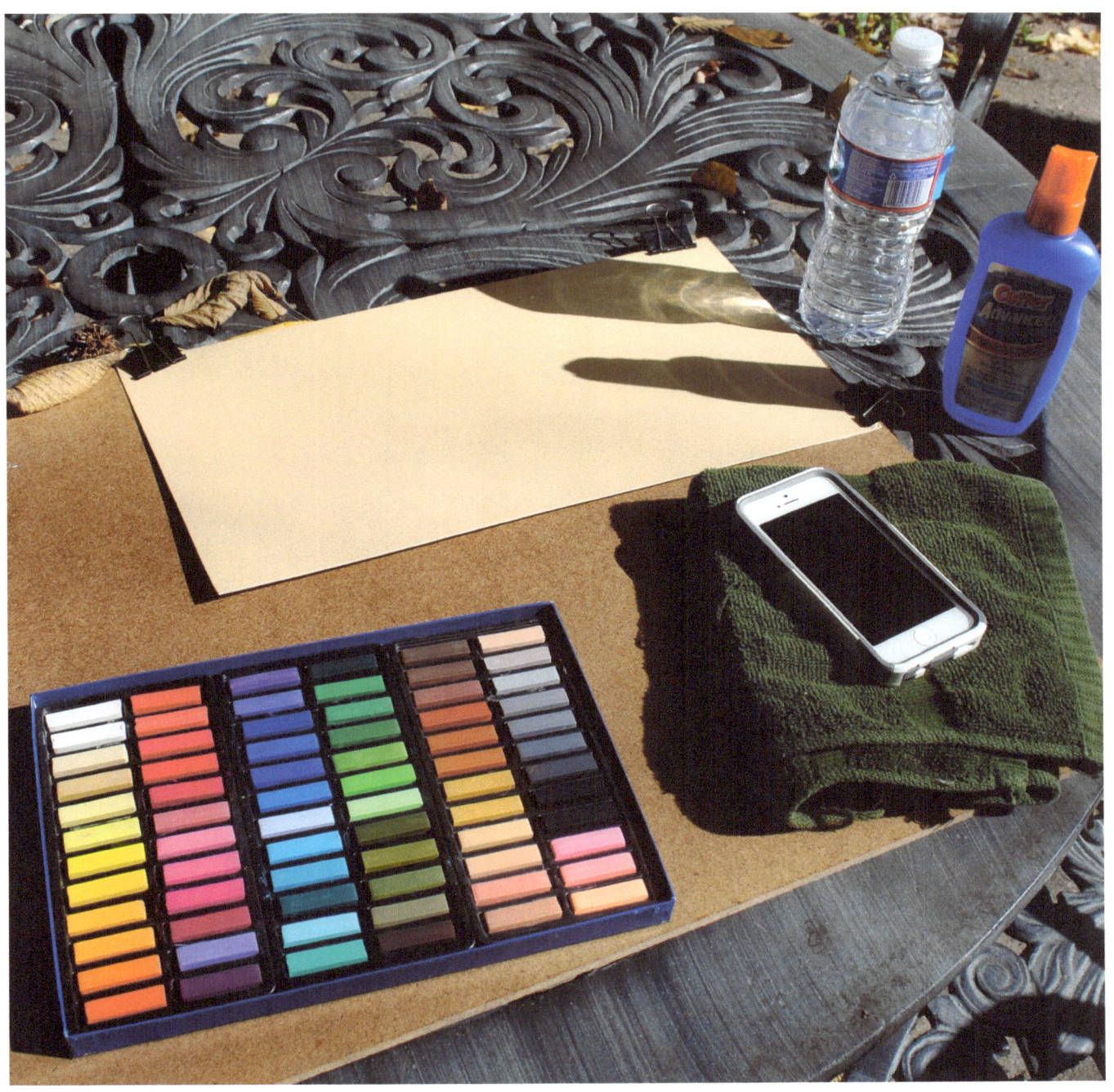

Pastel Papers and Additional Supplies

PastelMat has a finer surface on a sturdy card and comes in two paper pad sizes. The 12 in. x 16 in. is the most useful and not too large to carry in the field.

La Carte Pastel Card is offered in 14 colors. This is a textured card that you can cut to any size. You should start with smaller pieces of paper. La Carte also offers a pastel pad in a variety of colors. The downside to this paper is that it cannot get wet because the textured surface will be damaged.

Wallis Sanded Paper comes in two colors, white and Belgian mist. I prefer the flocked or sanded paper because it holds the pastels without spraying them with fixative. The sanded paper also reminds me of those early cave walls artists used before there was paper. A toned paper is helpful outside. White paper can be very bright.

UArt Sanded Paper is off-white and comes in a variety of seven different grades of grit.

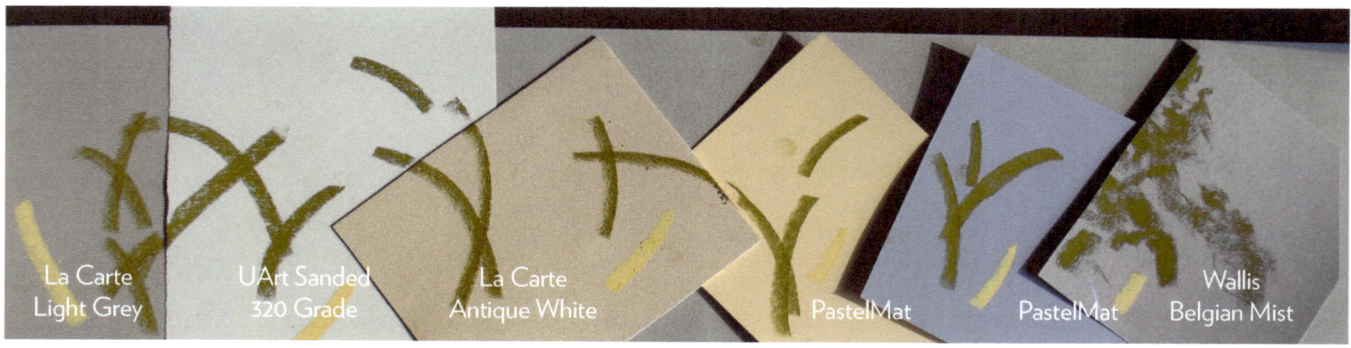

La Carte Light Grey | UArt Sanded 320 Grade | La Carte Antique White | PastelMat | PastelMat | Wallis Belgian Mist

A drawing board 18 in. x 18 in. is a good size for traveling and carrying out to the field. You can also use a piece of Masonite from the hardware store and add clips. Either is fine. A traditional art supply board has a hand hole to help you carry the board. This board will be your working surface on your lap, where you will clip your paper and set your pastel box.

A hand towel to place over your lap and wipe your hands and a ridged piece of **fine textured sponge.**

Additional items to include are this book, a folding chair, bug spray, tote bag, cell phone, and a bottle of water to drink or wash your fingers.

Thoughts on painting to consider...

1. Sit in the shade.

2. Observe the sun and the direction of shadows. Your view should have a variety of sun and shade.

3. Do not try to be too careful at first. Begin with a gesture drawing.

4. Look for basic shapes of colors and form, and block them into your gesture drawing.

5. The form of a maple tree is the same as an apple—a sphere with sunlight hitting on one side and shadow on the other. Look for basic shapes. See example below.

6. A dark value in the foreground will be a mid-value in the background.

7. Your foreground will have your darkest darks and lightest lights. These values will diminish as you recede into the distances. The colors become cooler, bluer.

8. Warm colors come forward, cool colors recede in the picture plane.

9. Do not try to copy colors with pastels out in the field. Pick a color that works for you and enjoy it.

10. Create your edges by the contour of your positive spaces (the leaf), as well as the contour of your negative spaces (the space between the leaves).

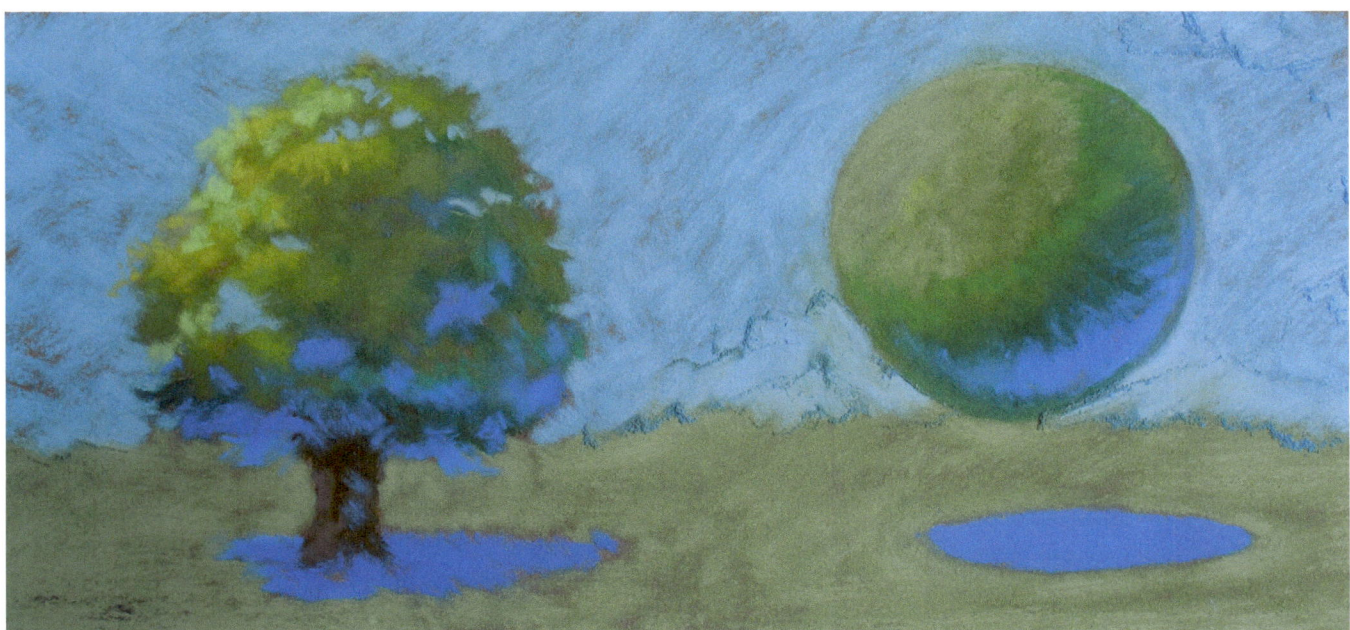

In the beginning, keep it simple and keep it small.

GESTURE DRAWING

Gesture drawing is traditionally a rapid drawing to study the human figure, its motion and form. I use it in the same way to study the landscape and the values of the landscape because these values can change instantly.

With one color, find your horizon and draw a line, the clumps of trees or features, areas of shade, and directional lines in your view.

Draw quickly. Do not deliberate over this in the beginning. The drawing should be an exploratory drawing. Your gesture drawing will prevent your landscape from being too stiff. You will cover it all up in the end, changing and refining, but it gives you placement.

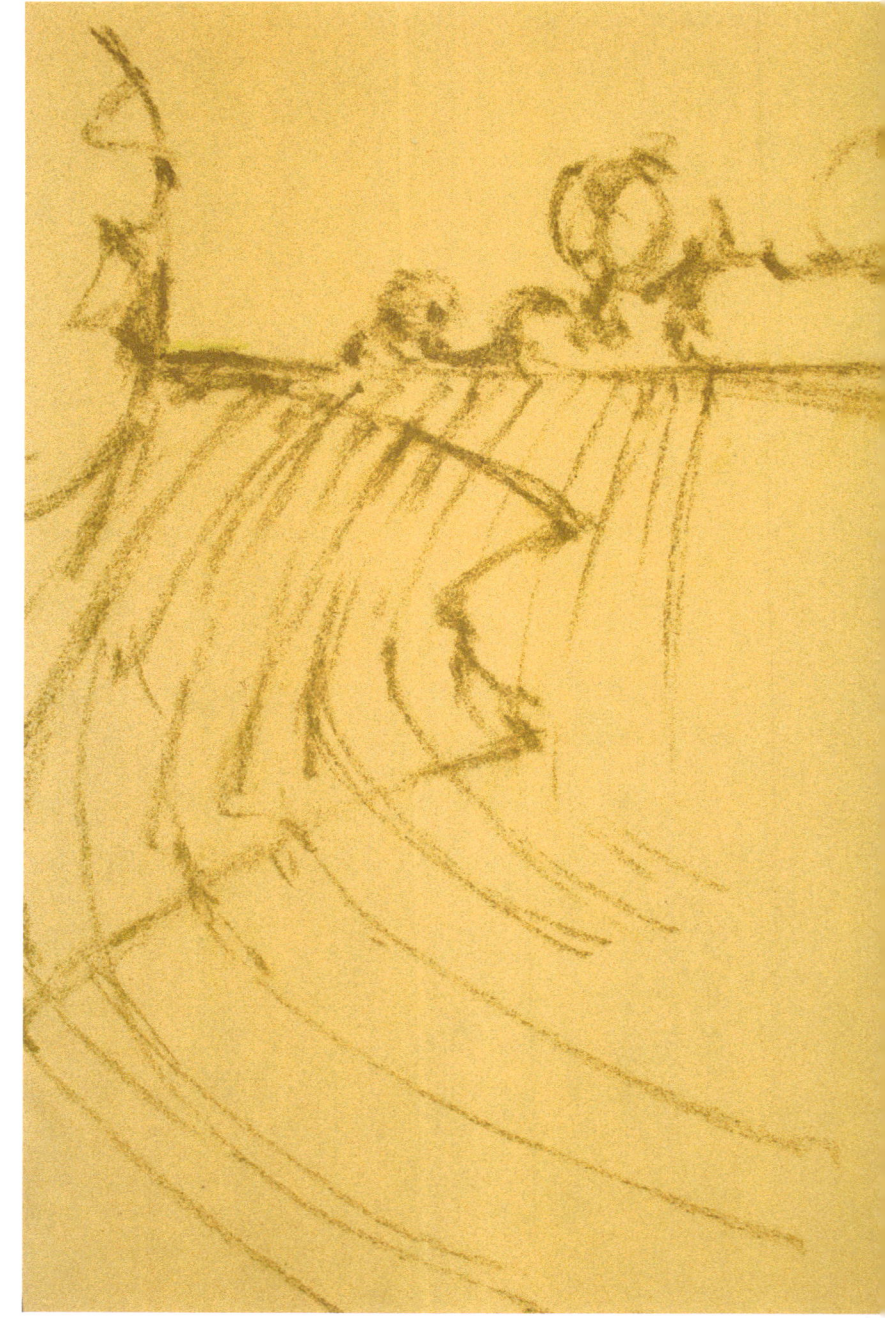

BLOCK IN THE DARKS

Blocking in the dark values is your next quick step. Squint at the landscape and see the darks as very basic shapes, and with no regard to what they are. They need to be just dark shapes with a definite form. Within this dark form, you may find trees and grass and roads, but not at first—just the dark shapes.

While out in the field, the sun and clouds can change rapidly. This gesture drawing of the darks (pictured right) can give you an anchor to keep you organized. One of the joys of painting in the field is the changing light. Since we are there to experience nature, we can observe the changes and include what we find stimulating. This is why working from a photo is not very interesting. In the end, your painting will be the sum of your experience, not a copy of the landscape.

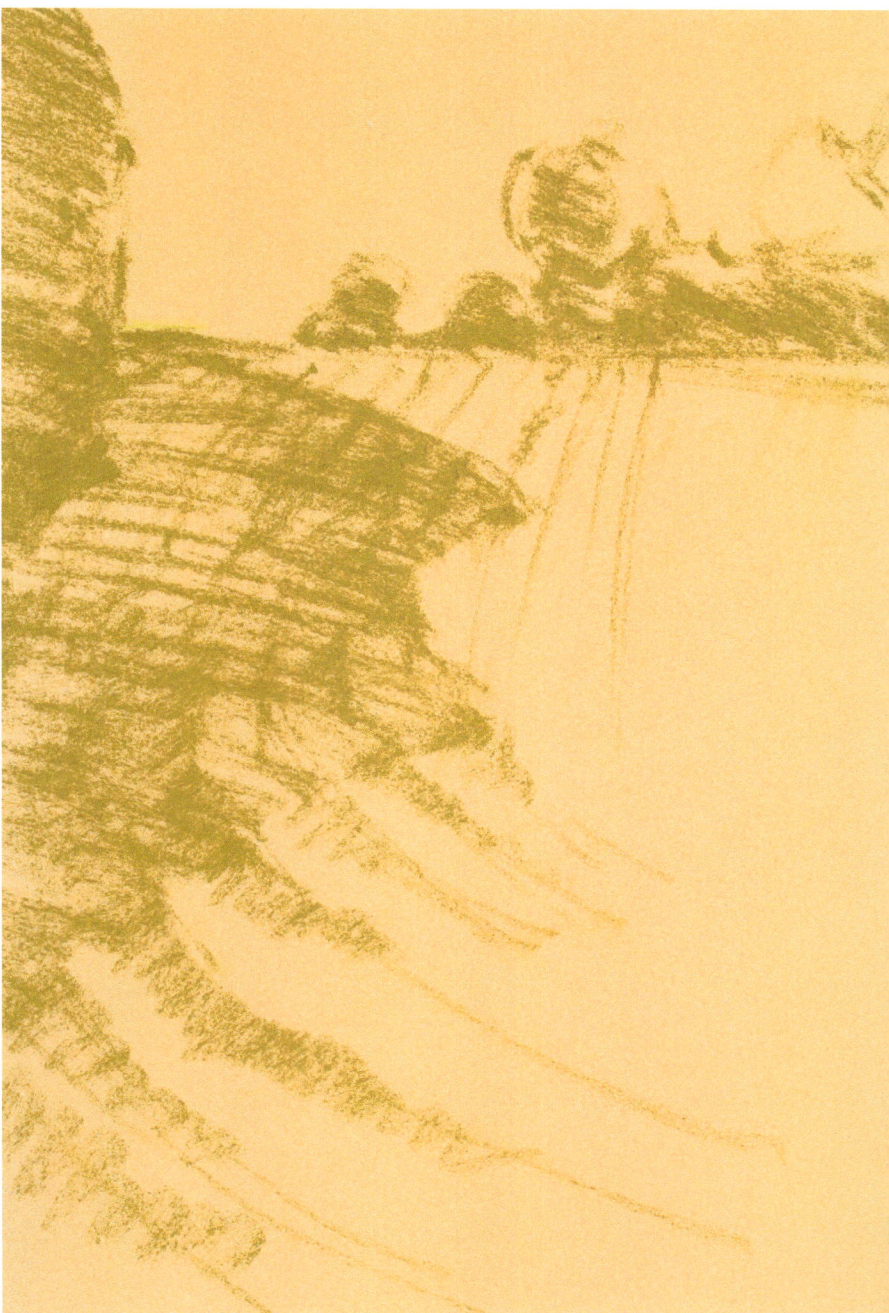

Explore the darks once more. Use your piece of sponge or packing foam to pull off the excess pigment and add to the study of your dark areas.

Whenever you get into a place you have built up with too much pigment and it is not working out, just clear the area with the sponge and rework it. There will always be a residue left behind but that is a useful undertone. Traditional erasers will not work on sanded or flocked paper.

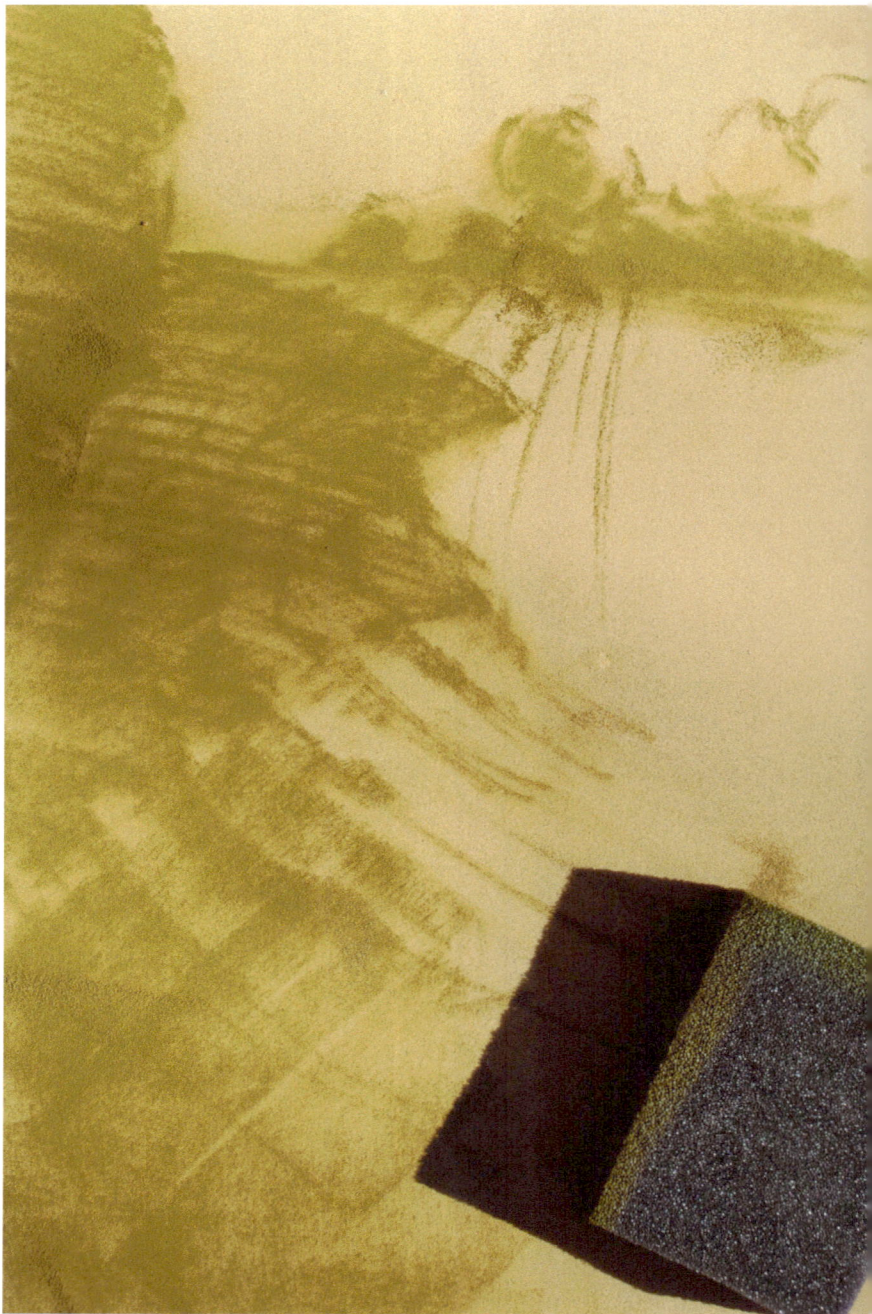

NEGATIVE SPACE

Negative space is the space between objects. In landscape painting, it can be the sky or earth but it is just as important as the subject or positive space. In this next observation, the sky that surrounds the trees in the distance is a light form and a negative space. I have used the sky color and form to redefine my trees, always exploring the edges—both drawing the form or trees and the space around the trees. In this example, drawing the form between the trees. This gives you two chances to explore nature and see it anew.

Continue to block in your lighter areas and begin to play with the color. You are on your own now to see the landscape.

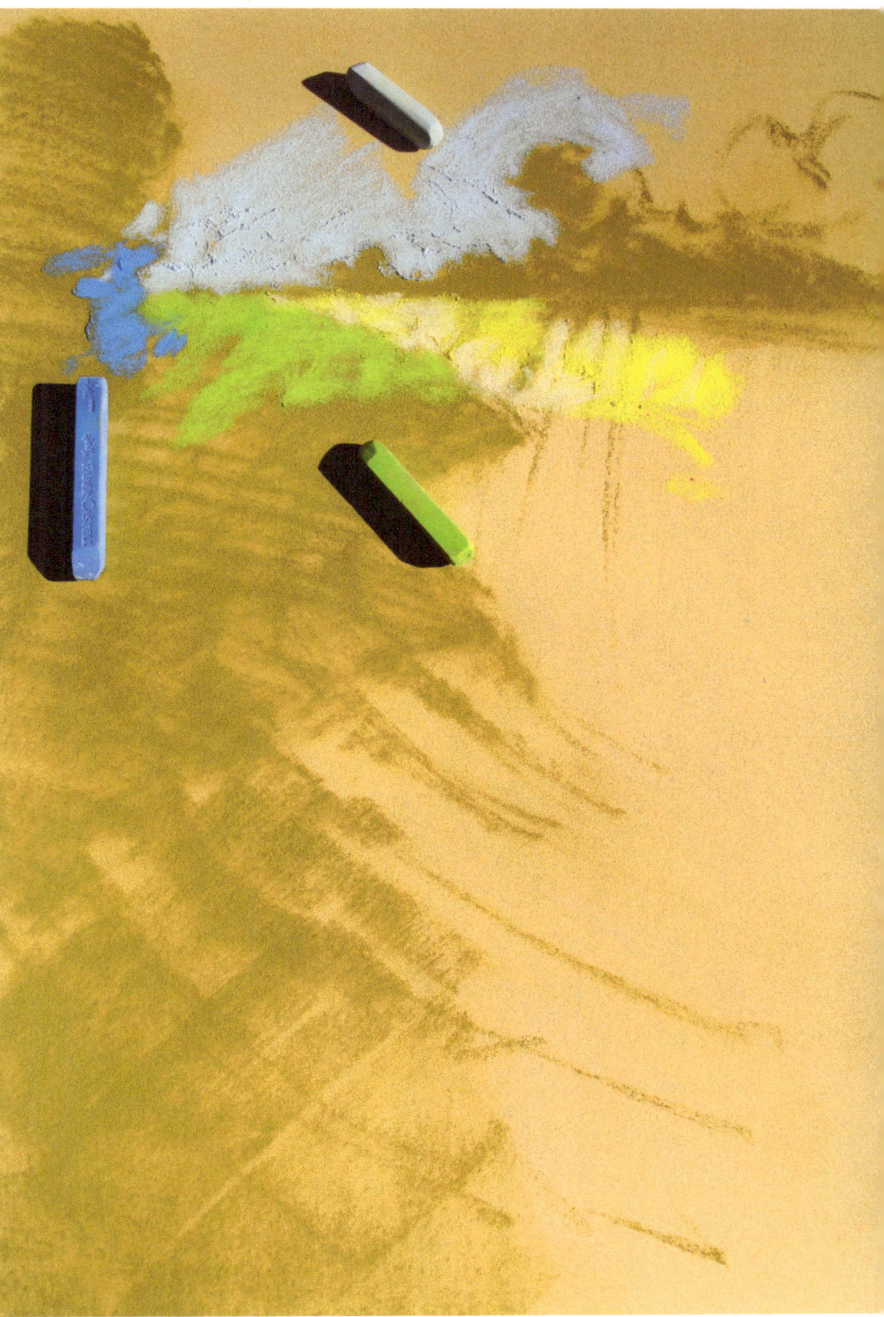

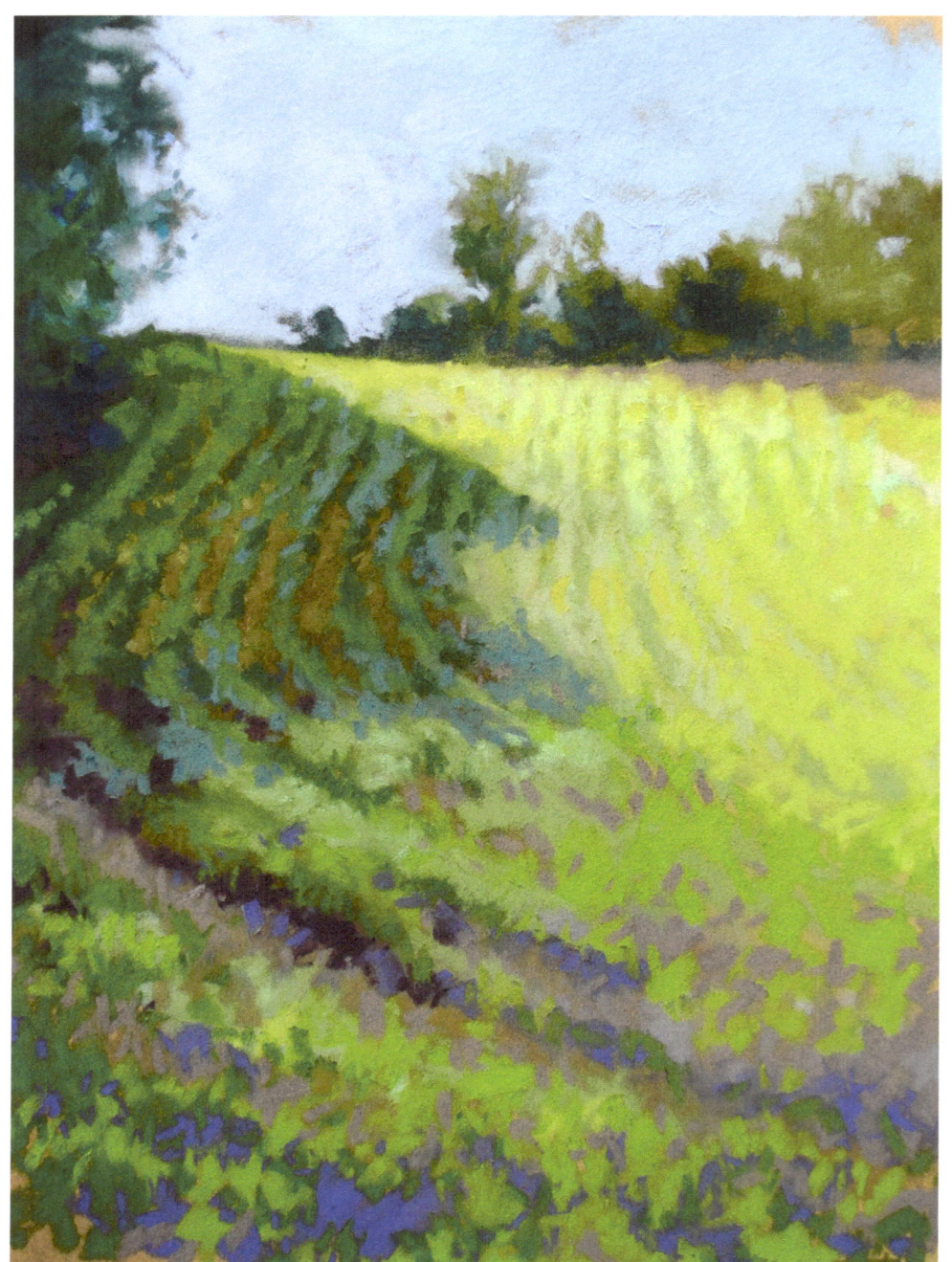

May Green, Pastel on La Carte Pastel Card, antique white, 11 in. x 15 in. by Alexia Scott, June 2013

Somehow this was a comfortable field. Driving from here to there in Maryland, I found two pastels waiting to happen.

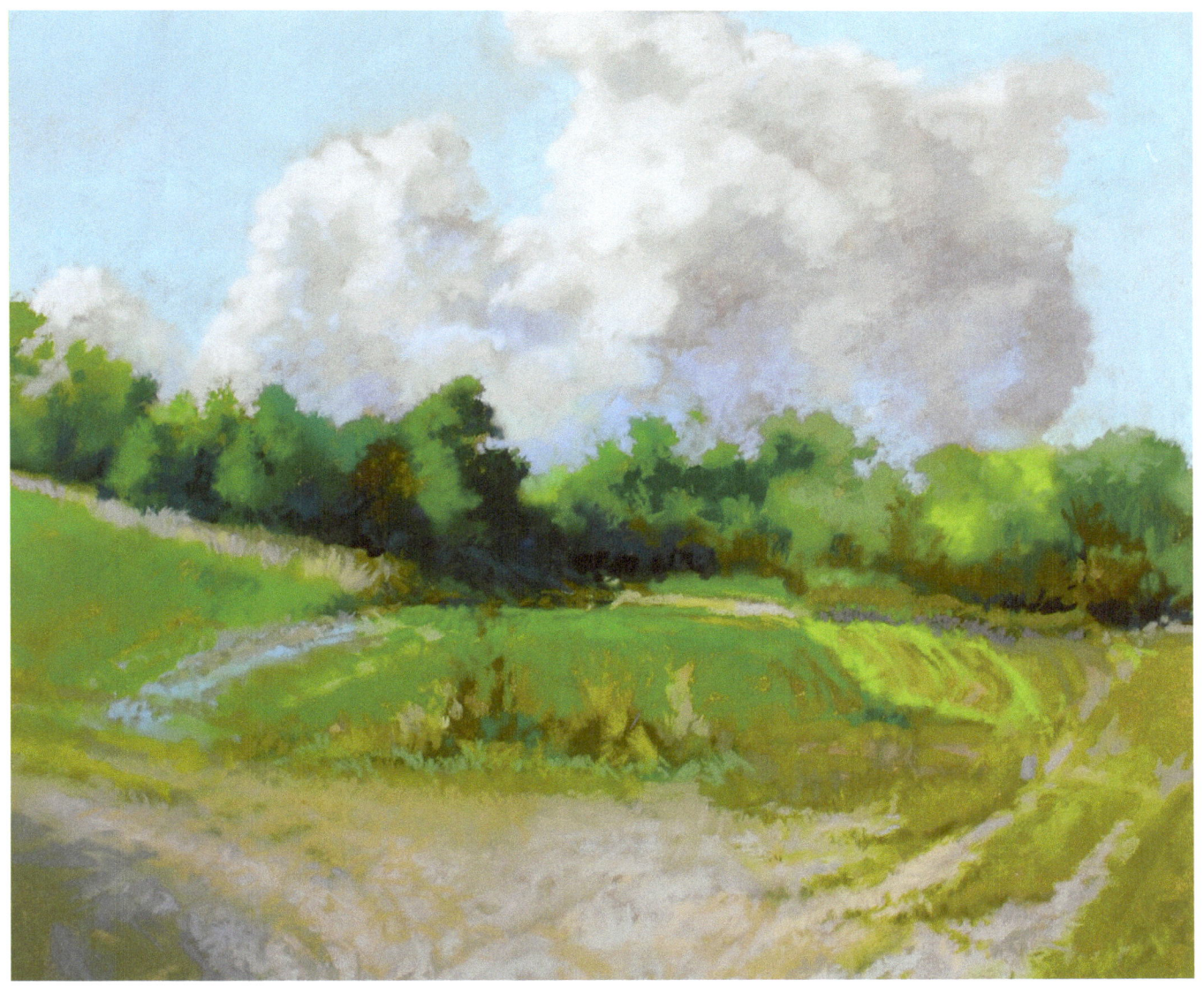

Field and Cloud, Pastel on La Carte Pastel Card, 24 in. x 24 in.
by Alexia Scott, July 2013

I love to paint a path or road. Growing up in the midwest, I would follow every path and road while exploring the landscapes. These two views were next to each other.

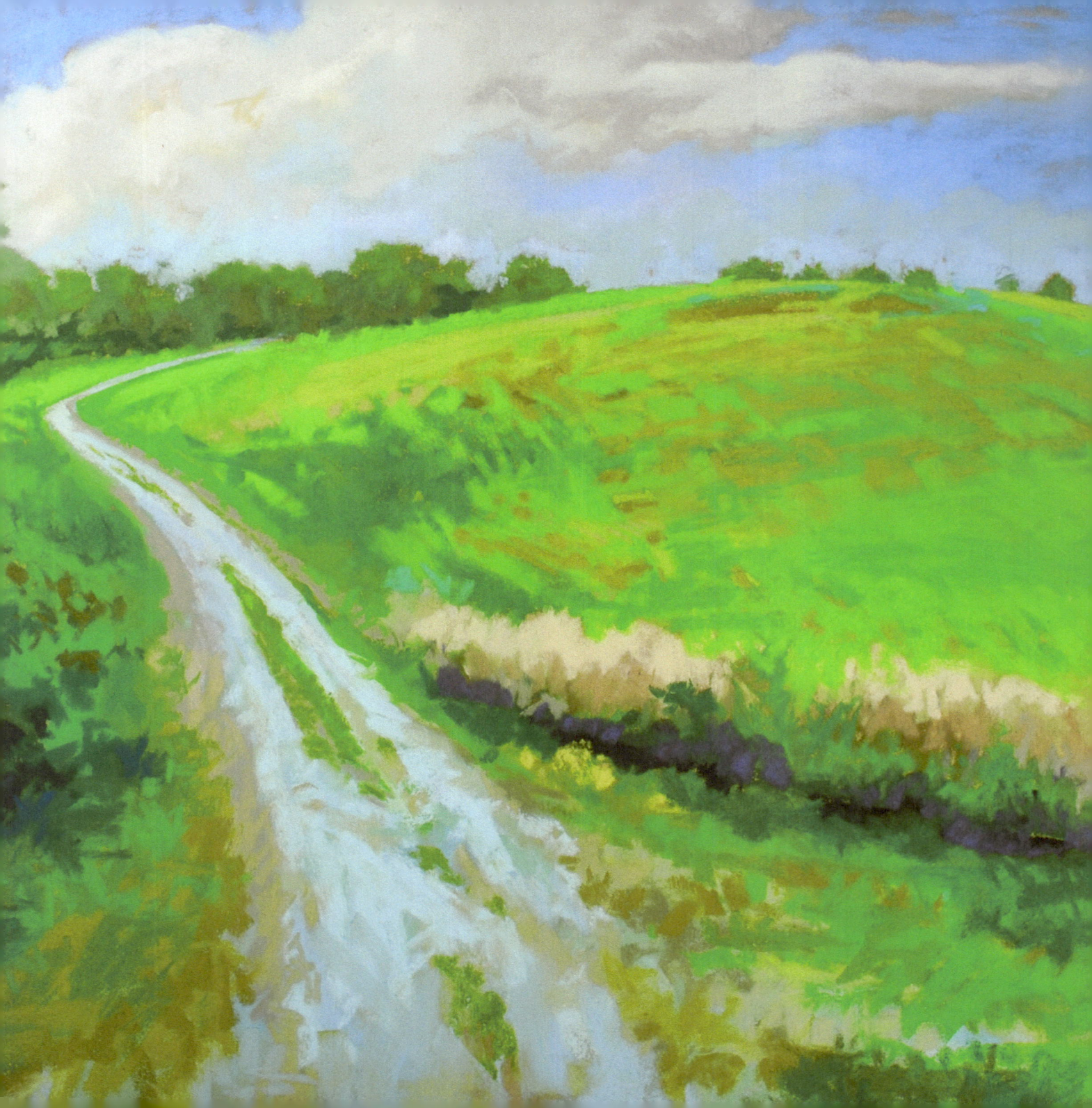

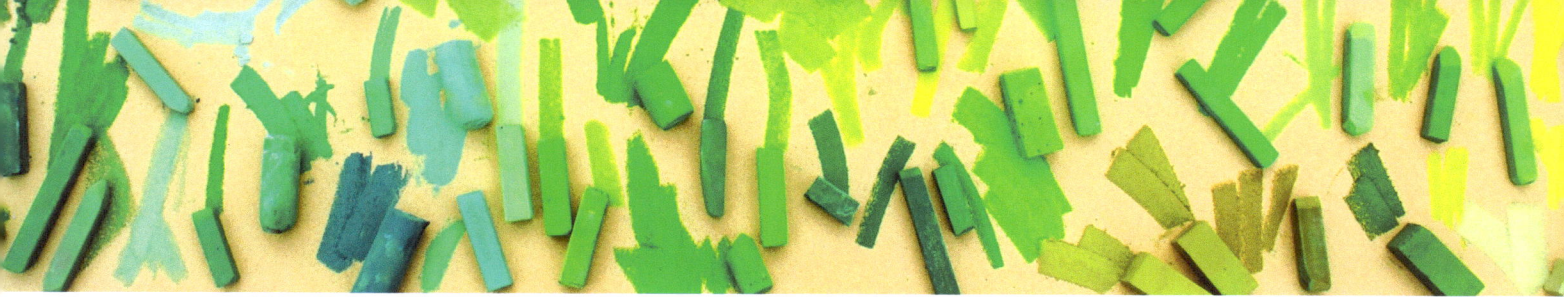

Green Pigments: Never too Many Green Pastels

All colors are exceptional and I am grateful that humans can process such an endless number of individual colors because all creatures cannot. Green is a particularly interesting color because, according to studies, we can see more shades of green than any other color. Green is the color of life, of new living things, and marks places where we find water—essential to our existence. Try switching to a green highlighter and see how much you enjoy it.

Green is a secondary color in art. It is created by mixing two primary colors: yellow and blue. This mixture creates a sliding scale of greens from yellowish greens to bluish greens, but what is the importance of the differences? Picture a Sugar Maple tree on a sunlit day in mid-summer...the tree is green but there are, in fact, hundreds of shades of green in a very subtle order. Think of the tree as a globe on a stick. The leaves closest to the sunlight will be a warm yellow green reflecting the yellow light of the sun. The leaves on the opposite side of the tree will be a slightly bluish green away from the light. Warmer greens (a bit of red in the mixture) create the appearance of the color coming forward to the eye, while cooler greens recede from your eyes.

This is a complex visual experience and a wonder of nature. Understanding what you are seeing allows you to be expressive. It is not necessary to copy the landscape, but to preserve the emotional beauty of nature and your experience.

Left Image: *Just Off Route 17*, Pastel on La Carte Pastel Card, 16 in. x 18 in.
by Alexia Scott, July 2013

Virginia is very green. The rain and humidity can change a garden into a vine patch in a week, but it is a beautiful place to paint.

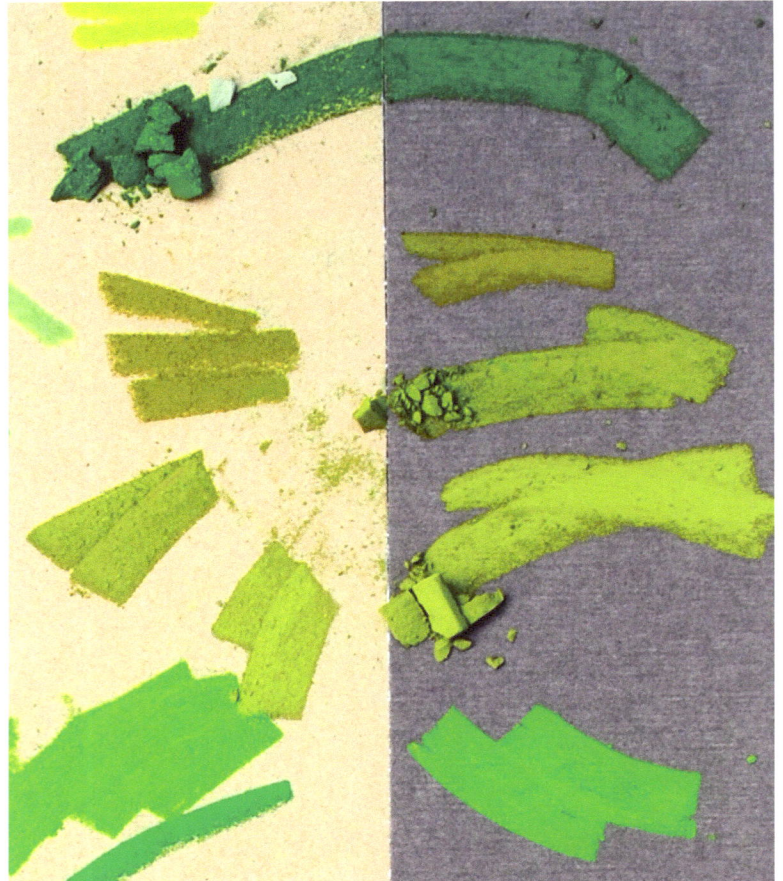

ALL COLORS ARE RELATIVE TO THEIR SURROUNDINGS

In pastel painting, we have the option of using a variety of colored papers which are referred to as grounds. On a darker ground, such as the Wallis Belgian mist, a mid-tone green pastel can look very light. I use the darker ground when I am painting a subject with very little sky and a lighter ground when I have more sky or clouds in my view. Pastels are opaque pure pigment, therefore, the ground color does not alter the pigment color in the same way a toned ground will alter an oil painting with translucent oil paints. However, the optical appearance can change the pigment a great deal. The individual pigment will change its appearance as you create your composition.

Generally, all pigment materials are the same and it is the binder that makes the difference between a pastel, an oil painting, watercolors, and the rest. The same red earth used in early cave paintings is used to form a red earth pastel. When mixed with Linseed oil, it becomes an oil paint. When mixed with gum Arabic, it becomes a watercolor. When you are working with pastels, you are using the pigment in its purest form. This natural state is what makes it a perfect media for work in the field.

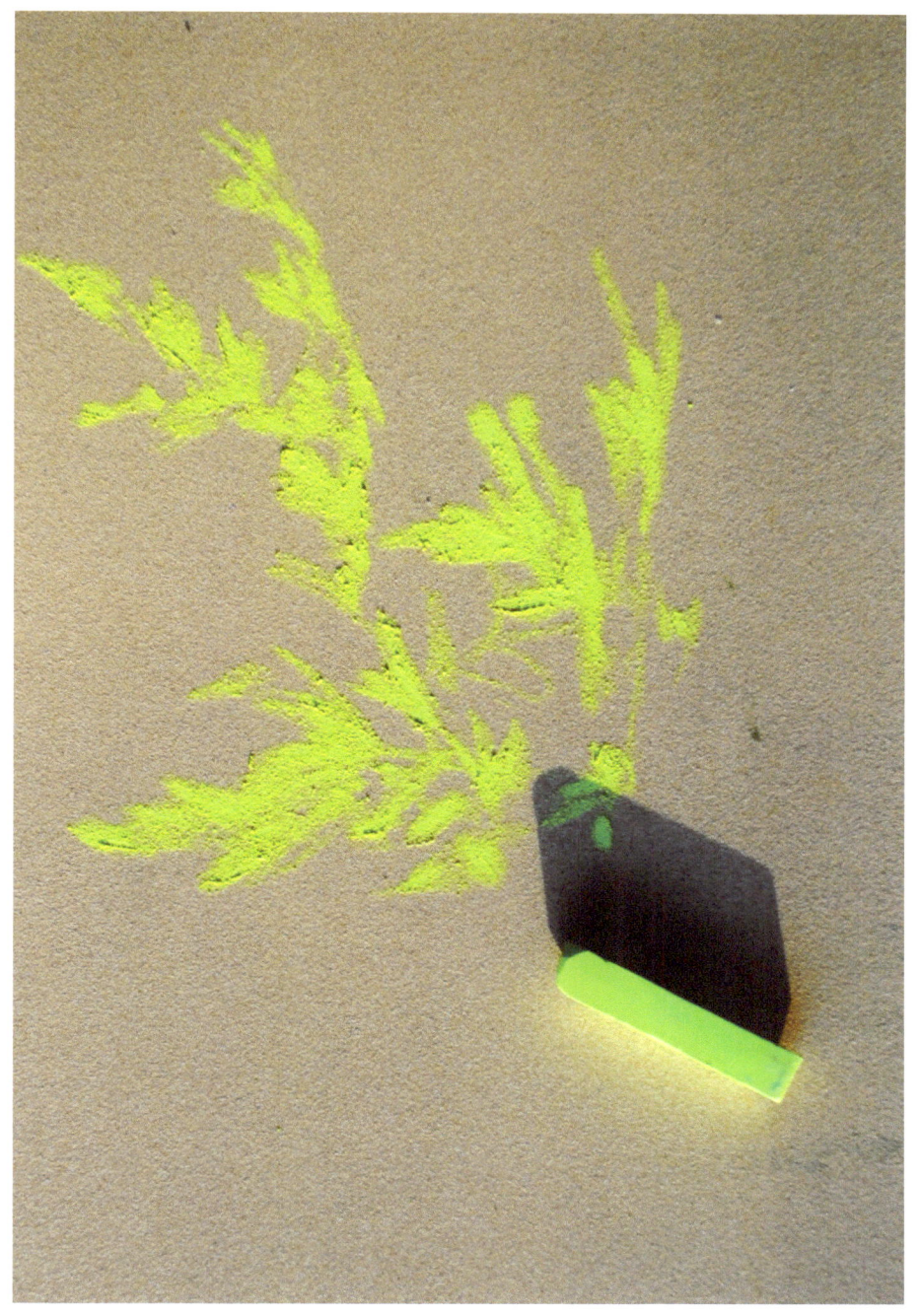

The green bush is never just green. While drawing a plant near my front door, I will need to draw fast. The sun is low creating long shadows and strong highlights. I choose a green to represent the leaves touched by the sunlight (pictured left). Notice the change in the appearance of the green in the shadow. Without the afternoon warm sunlight, the same green is a cooler green. The light creates the difference in color.

Colors change their appearance when viewed in sunlight to shade, and from outside in the field to inside the home. Many artists, including the Impressionists, work on their paintings in both plein air and in the studio, in order to achieve the desired colors for the painting.

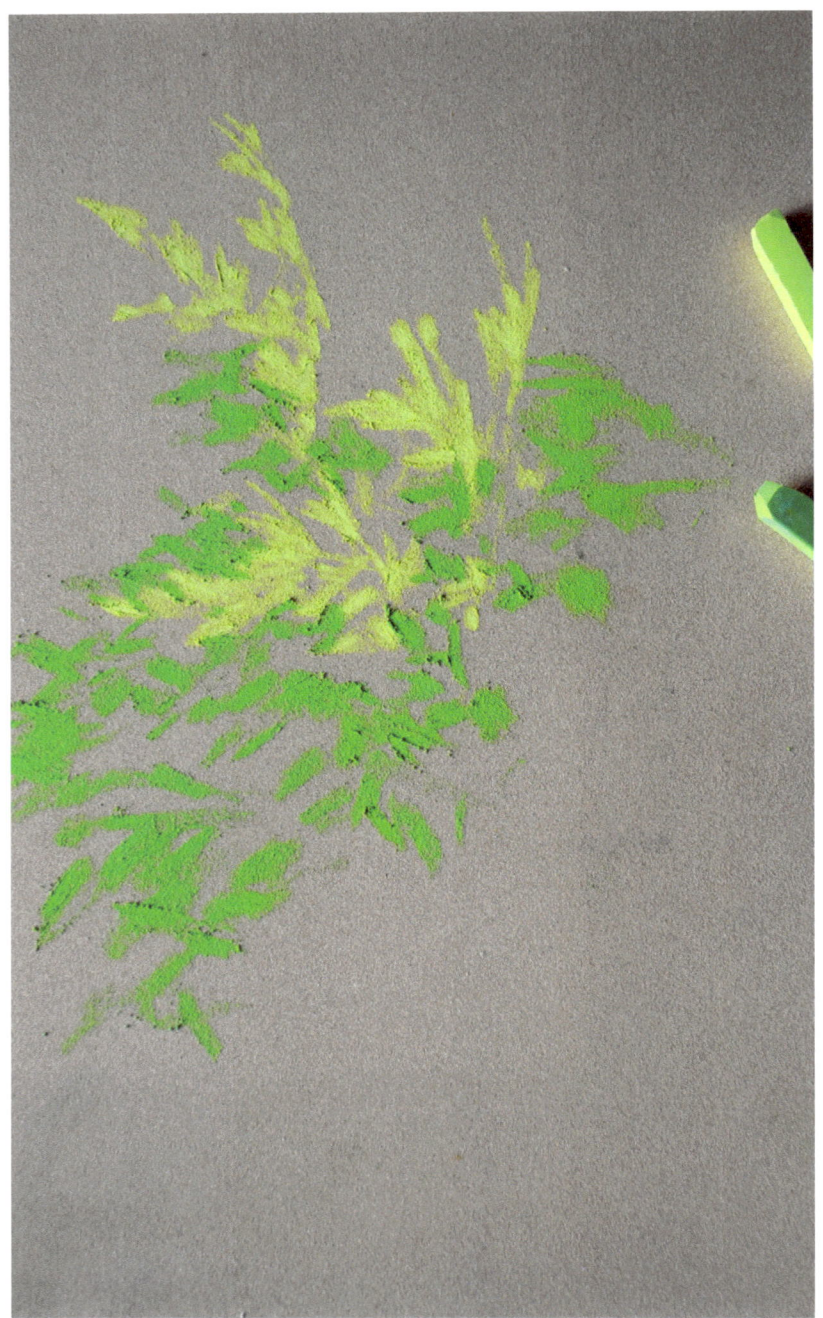

Working fast to catch the light, I choose my middle green. This is the base green for the plant. This green is in daylight but no direct sunlight touches this area. I do not draw the leaves, but make marks resembling the movement of the leaves. I am working from sunlight into shadow, from outside the plant to inside the plant. This clear true green is the primary green color of my overall composition. Whether I truly see this color in this plant or not, I choose to use it and relate the other colors of the composition to this color. I am using the plant as my guide.

This is an 8 in. x 10 in. painting on La Carte Pastel Card, antique white. As I photograph my drawing, the changing light changes the paper color but it is all the same drawing.

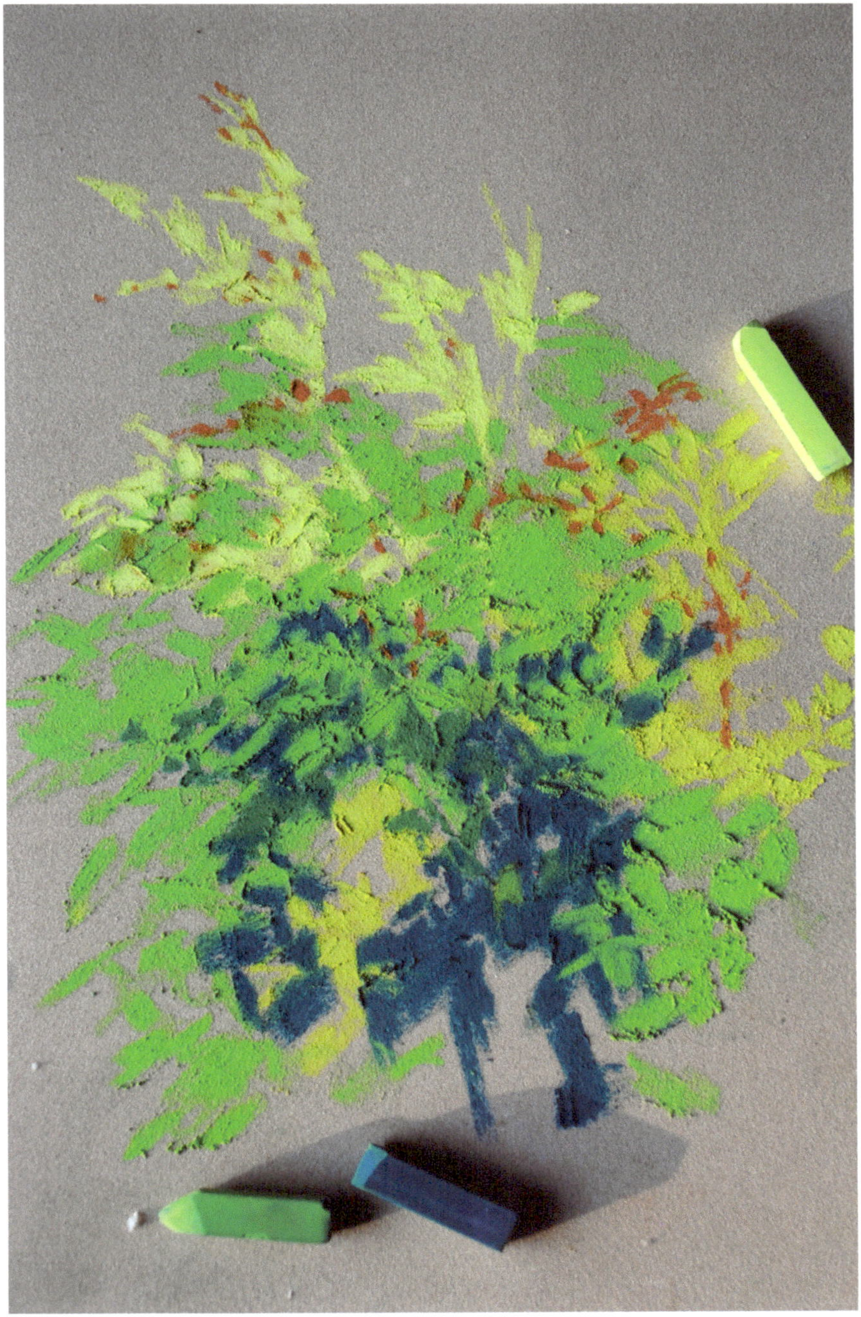

Using a cooler blue green, I begin to work down into the plant where the plant shadows its own leaves. Here you will find many greens and areas where the lighter sunlit green peeks through. All areas painted with the same pastel color will appear at the same distance from your eye.

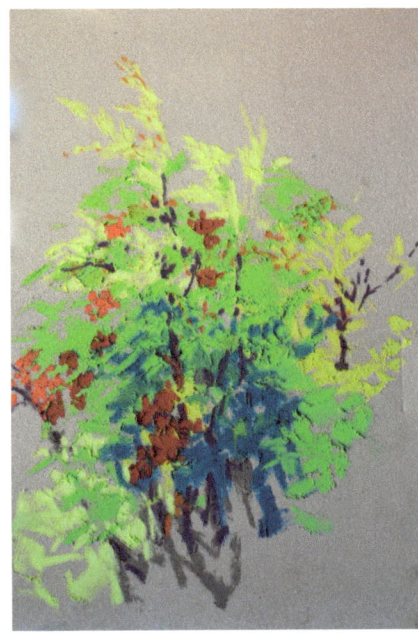

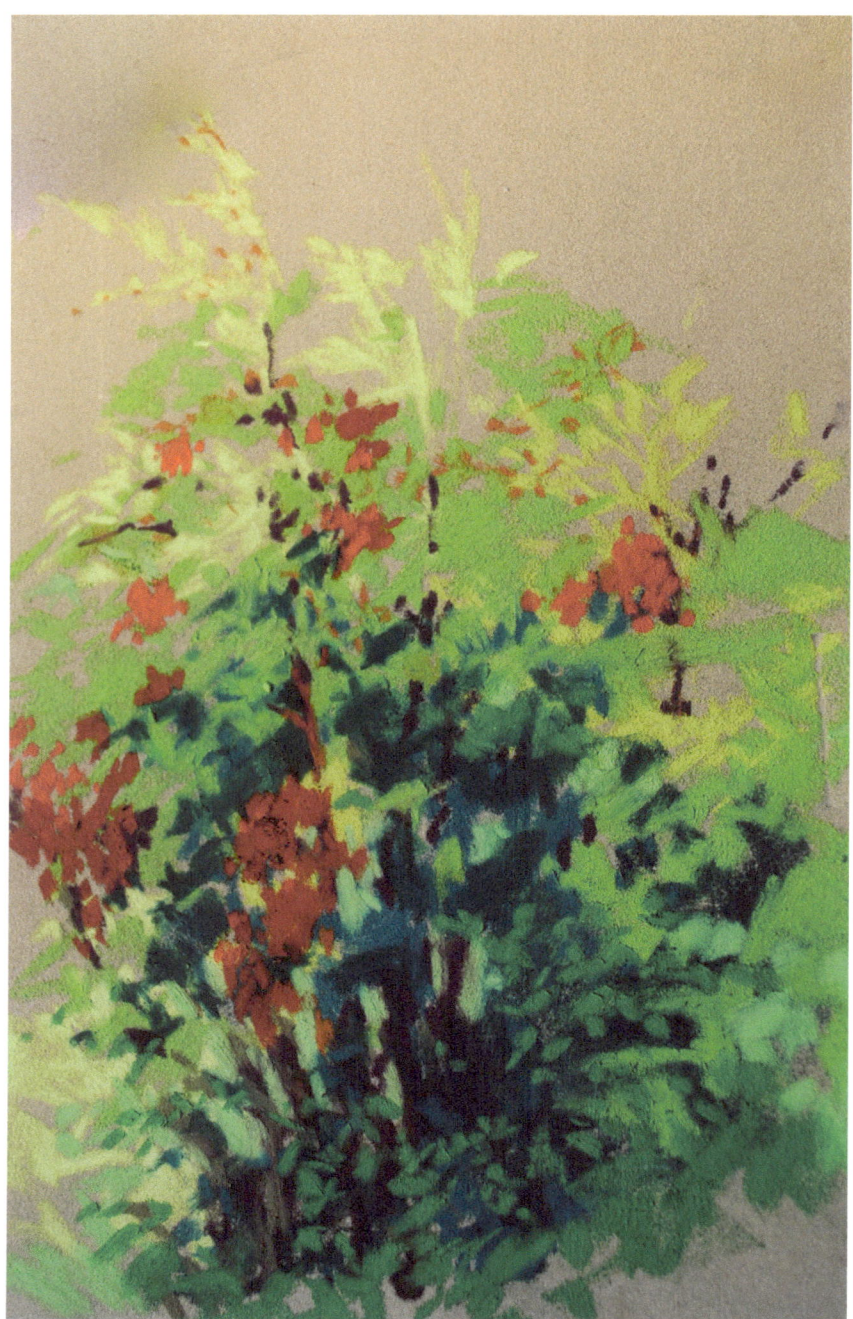

As I work into the darker areas of the plant, my eyes adjust to the darker area. This can fool you into misreading the dark values making them too light and competing with the sunlit areas. This will flatten the look of the subject if you are not careful. To avoid this pitfall, I continually look at the whole subject to observe the darks and lights relative to the whole plant.

Pastels can draw on top of other pastel marks, but if you get too much of a buildup you may have a mess. Remember to use the sponge to pull off unwanted buildup and also tone an area.

At this point in my small study, I am content with the results but I think I will go a step further and place the "Green Plant" within its environment.

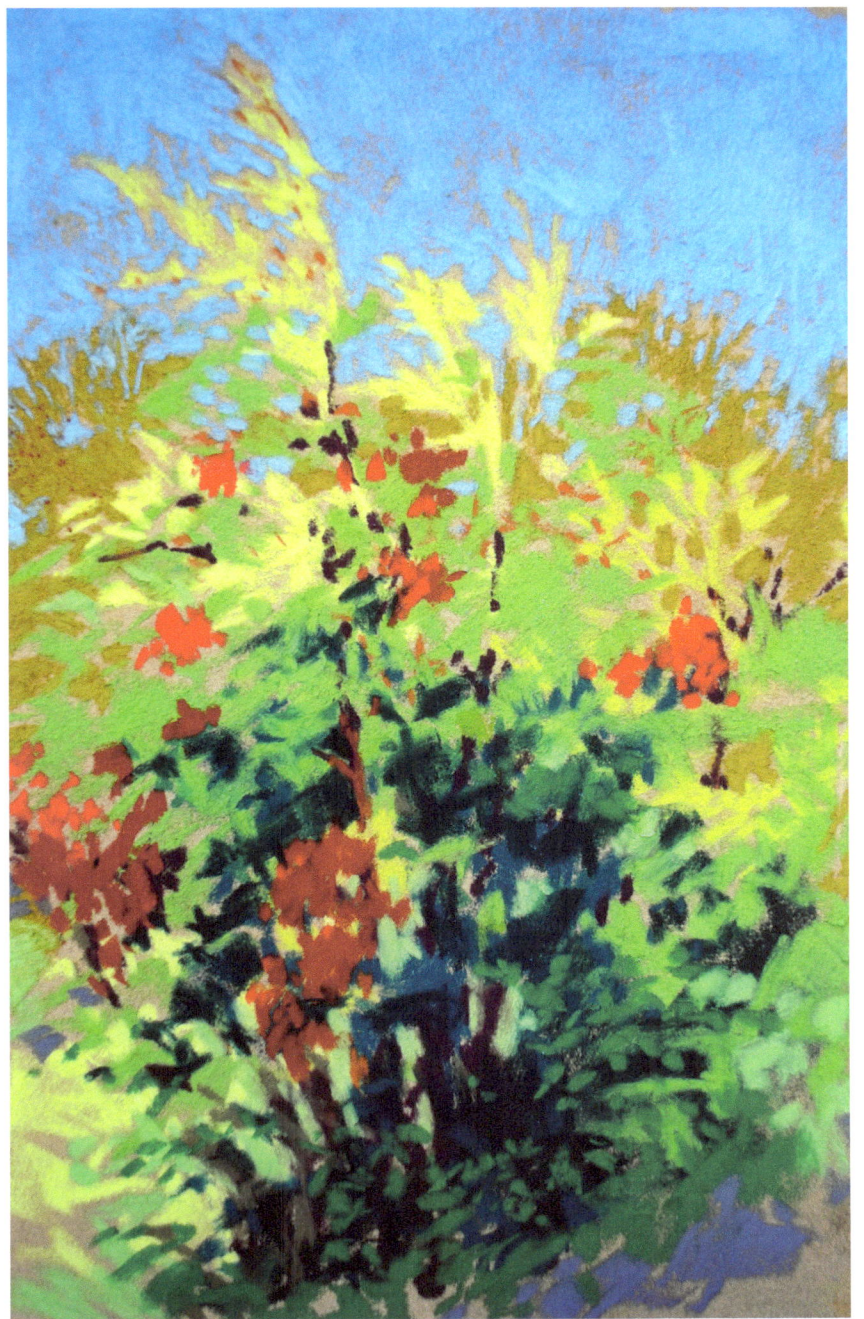

Before I lose the sun, I add the suggestion of the distant bare trees with the warm setting sun touching the branches. The sky is clear of clouds and I add the blue sky to bring out the lighter top of the bush. I find this to be a delicate process because it changes all the color relationships. There is also the problem of not having the pastel you need for the sky. My blue sky color is not just what I wanted, but what I had.

We have been exploring green and its many variations on a simple shrub, using a small selection of pastels from the Fiber–Castell set of Half Sticks.

A Green Plant, Pastel
by Alexia Scott, December 2013

AUGUST 2013—CALIFORNIA'S REDWOOD NATIONAL PARK

The Emerald Forest Campground and cabins in Trinidad, CA, are just outside Redwood National Park. The cabins are clustered in a beautiful grove of Coastal Redwoods and is a unique place to stay, paint, and wander among the trees. The cabins are clean and cozy and the town down the road has great coastal views and dining options. I am particularly fond of lodging locations where I can just step out the door and start painting.

Looking up in the morning from our cabin porch in the Redwoods, I was overwhelmed with the majestic trees. How would you even begin to study them and illustrate what you saw? I hoped to do a larger painting once back in Virginia, so I needed to learn the visual language of these trees. As the sun first touched the canopy, I began to draw on my small 8 in. x 9 in. paper. To suggest the massive structure, I chose to push the tree foliage against all sides of my picture plane edges, as though it would not fit. The fact that I was on the ground looking up also added to the illusion of greatness. In the movies, this is the way they filmed John Wayne to suggest his bold and heroic image. We all understand visual language, we just do not know we do.

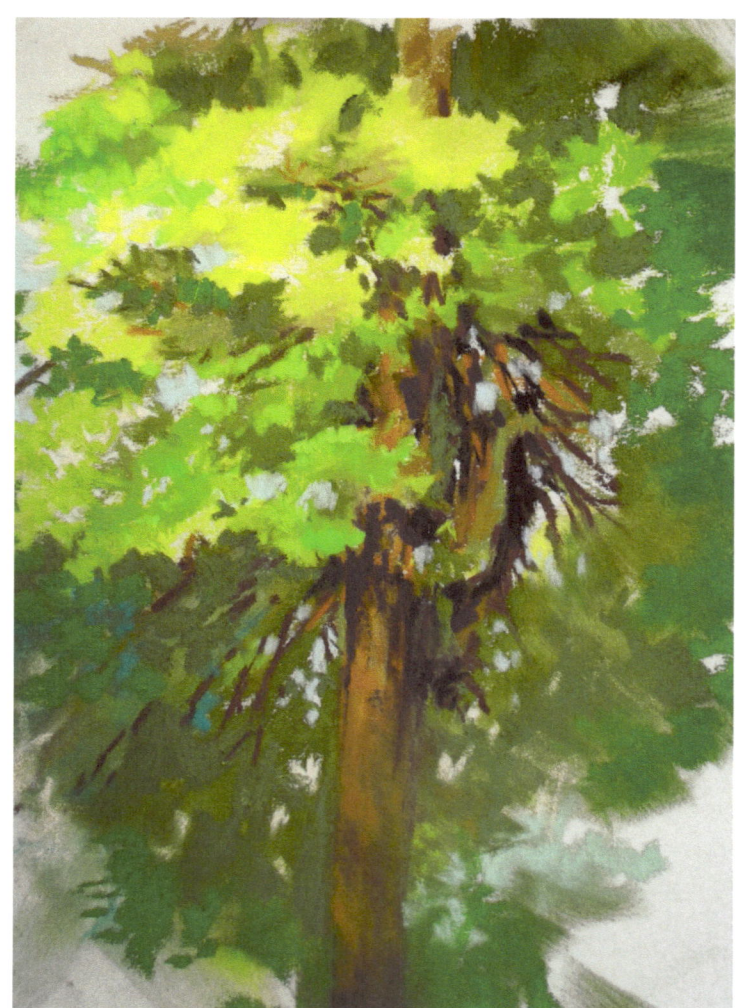

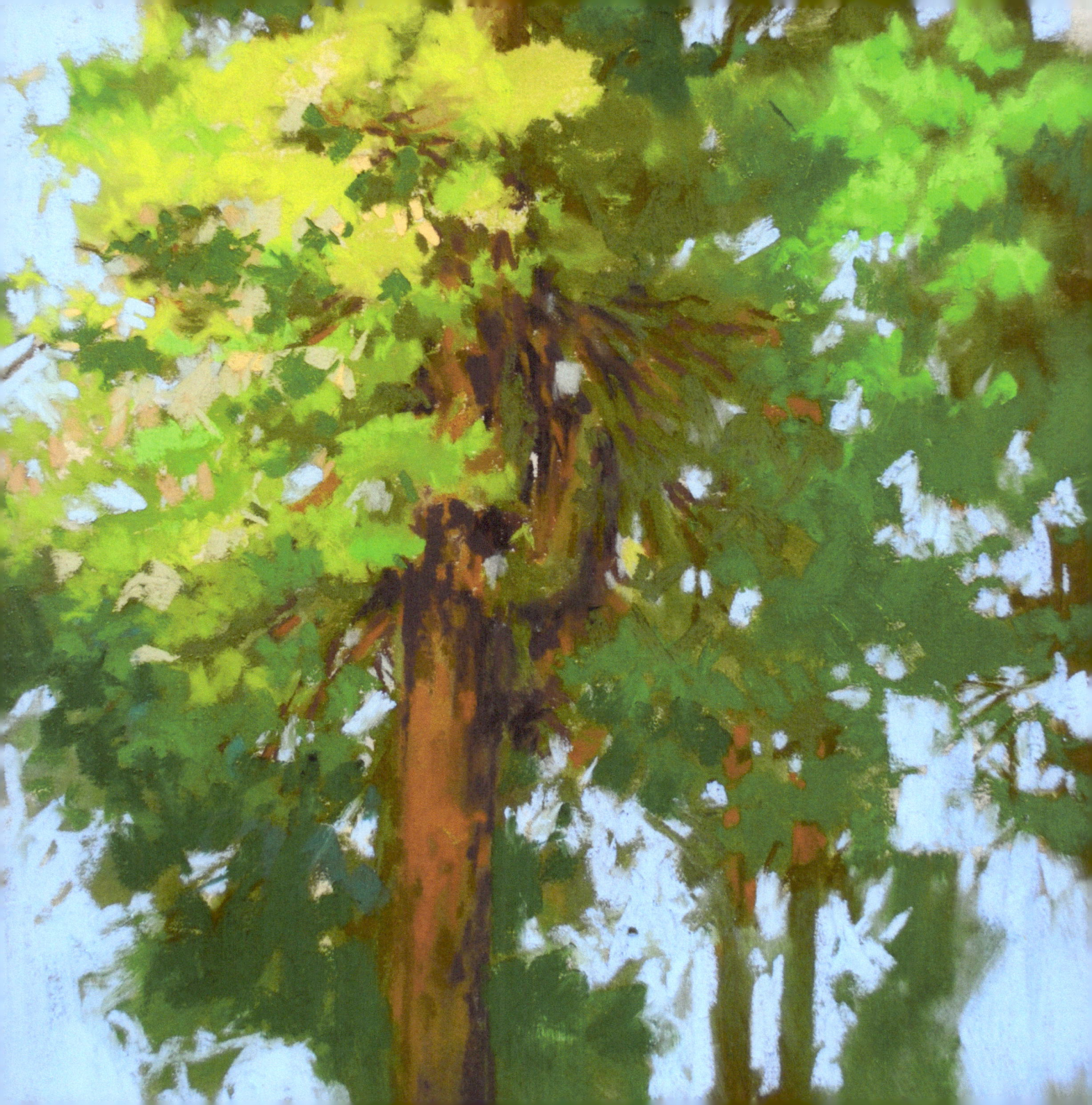

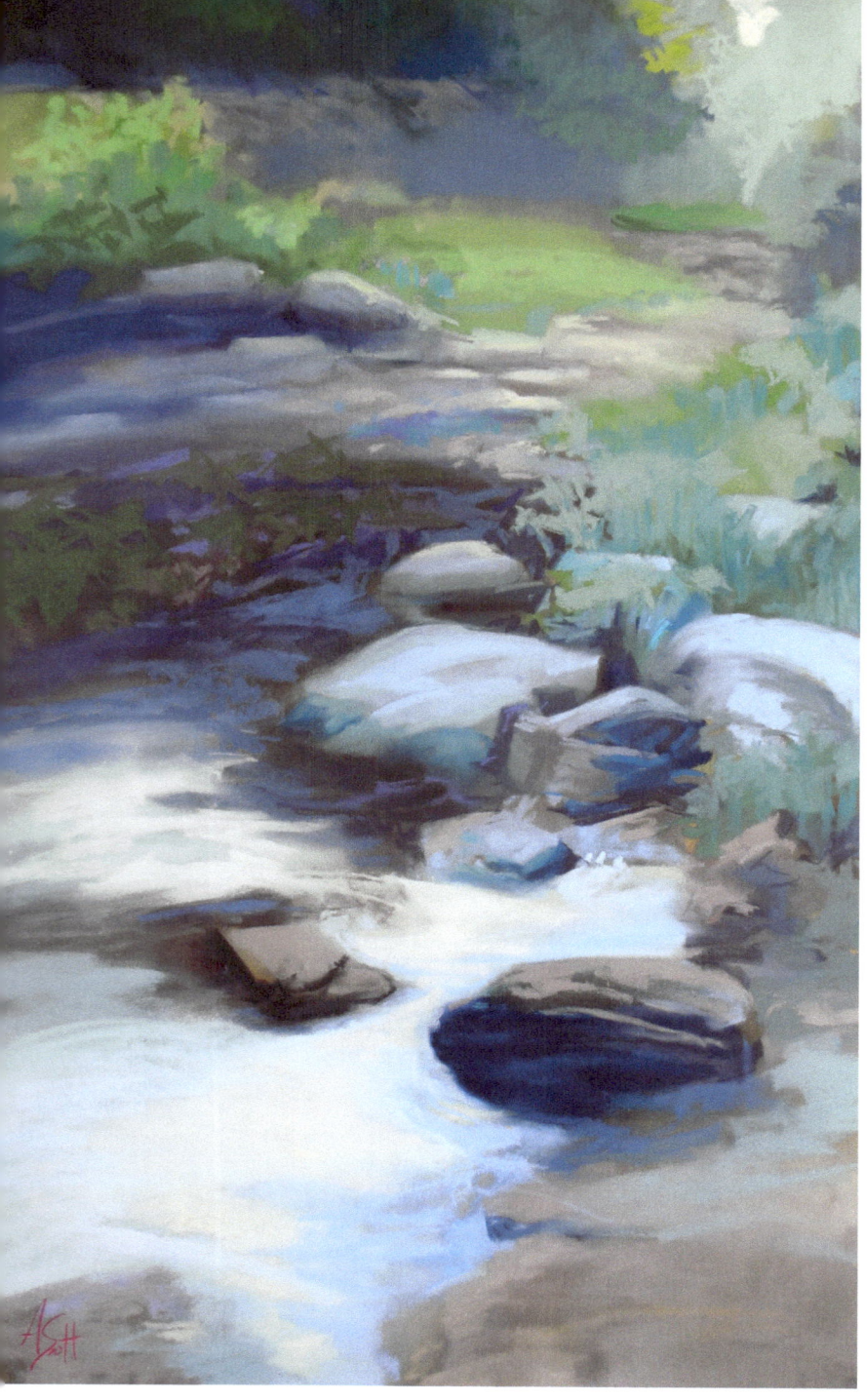

Deep Space

The pastel painting on the left is the canal at Great Falls National Park. This is a place I frequently paint and am able to take a full-size piece of pastel paper and work larger. At times, I return to complete the painting. This work is on a full-size piece of Wallis sanded paper in white, 24 in. x 36 in. I chose to use white because I knew I would be in the shade and that was what I had in the car. Remember the painting experience is not about your supplies, but about your time spent connecting with nature.

Rocks and Water, **Pastel, 24 in. x 35 in.**
by Alexia Scott

I started this on location in the summer, but the bugs drove me back to the studio.

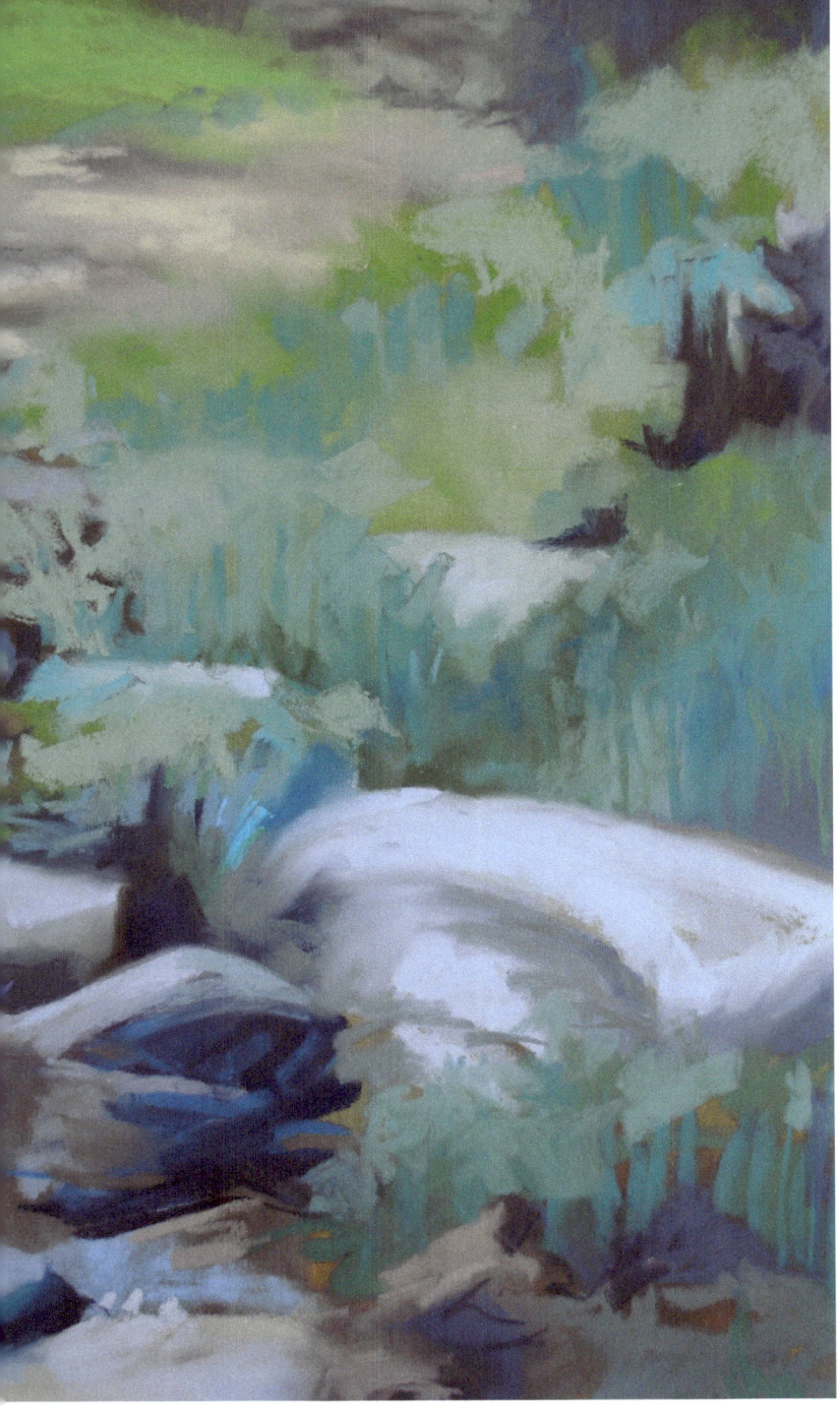

To create the illusion of deep space on a flat piece of paper, it is helpful to divide your view into three areas: foreground, middle ground, and background. Each of these areas can be handled by changing the values slightly and the scale of the objects. As you move back in space, your values diminish as well as the detail. In the foreground, your darks are the darkest and lights the lightest. Each step back pulls this value scale tighter. In the distance, no darks should be as dark as the foreground darks. A road, stream, or path will lead your eye into the distant plane. Colors become cooler due to atmospheric perspective as they move back in space and detail should be less. In the pastel of the canal, I added a detail of the middle ground. This was my focus for the painting. This is where I began to paint and subordinated all the other areas to this area.

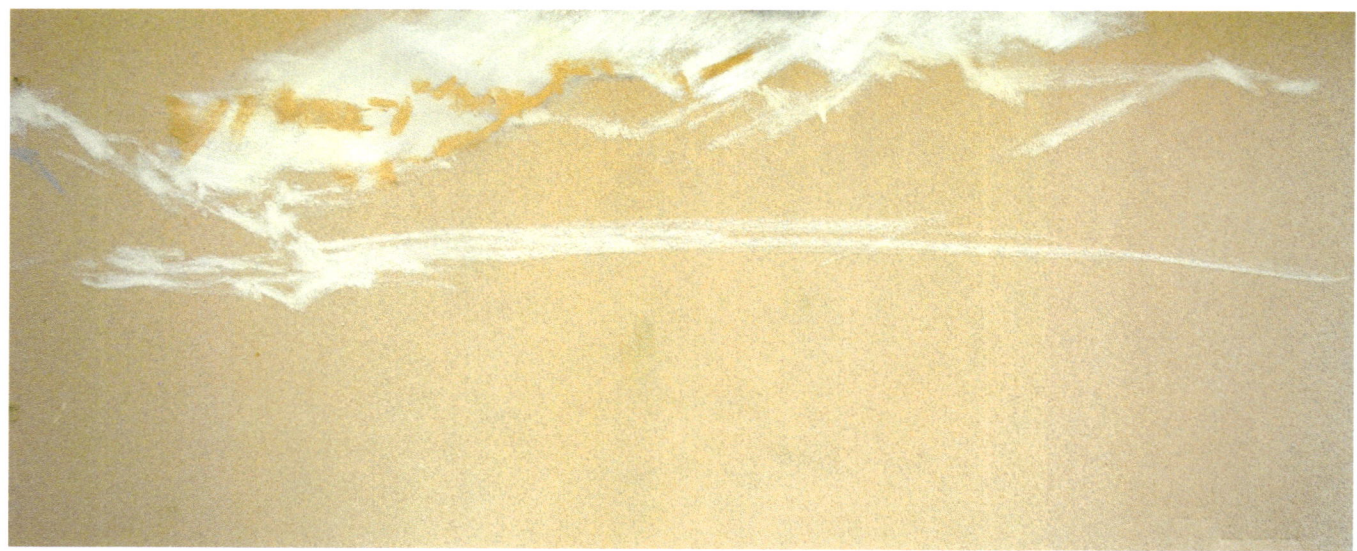

AUGUST 2013—CRATER LAKE, OREGON

The idea for this trip was to paint Crater Lake's bright blue water, but that did not happen. The closer we came to the park, the smokier the atmosphere became. While this did provide for some beautiful views, we did not see blue water. Since the water is a reflection of the sky, the water looked like smoke. There were many forest fires raging to the east. We were hoping for some rain until the park ranger remarked there would only be more lightning strikes and more fires. I painted this view sitting at an open window in the lodge on the third floor. It is the view to the back of Crater Lake Lodge.

I begin by finding the back edge of my middle ground. This is not always where to begin, but it helps keep you oriented. It is helpful to remember that you do not want any extreme detail beyond that point. The sun is just emerging from the left and I am working on La Carte Pastel Card, antique white, 7 in. x 17 in. When I travel, I toss all my odd leftover pieces of pastel paper in my case.

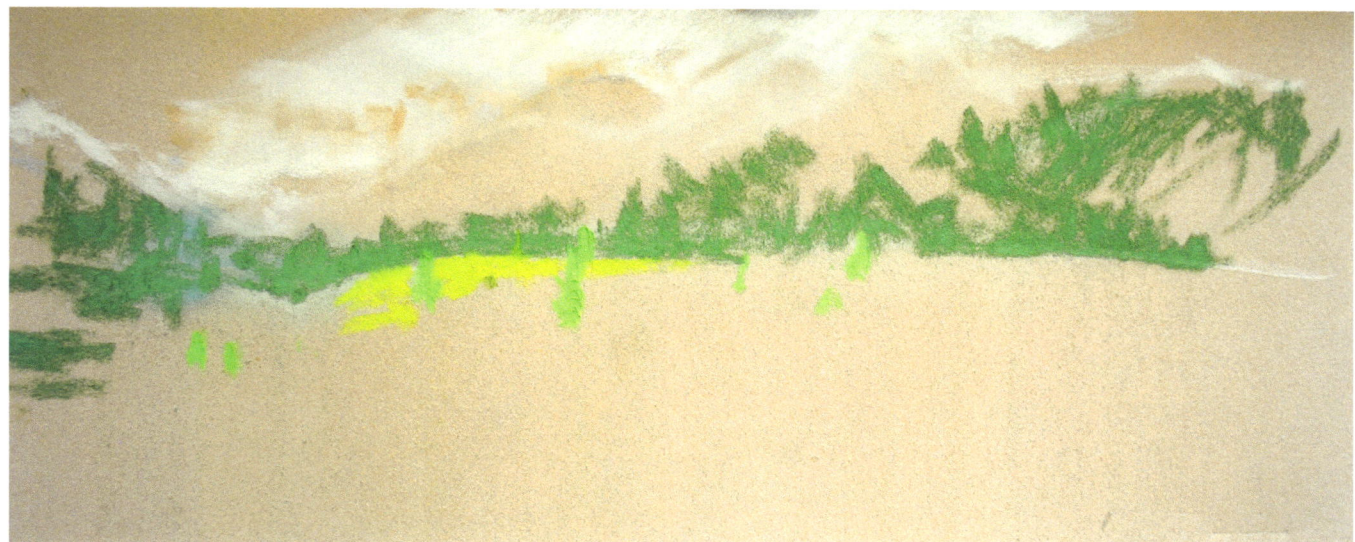

The sun seems to be arriving through a space in the mountains. The trees and middle ground are its first subjects. I enjoy my painting in its earliest stage, but I am there to watch and experience the event, so I continue.

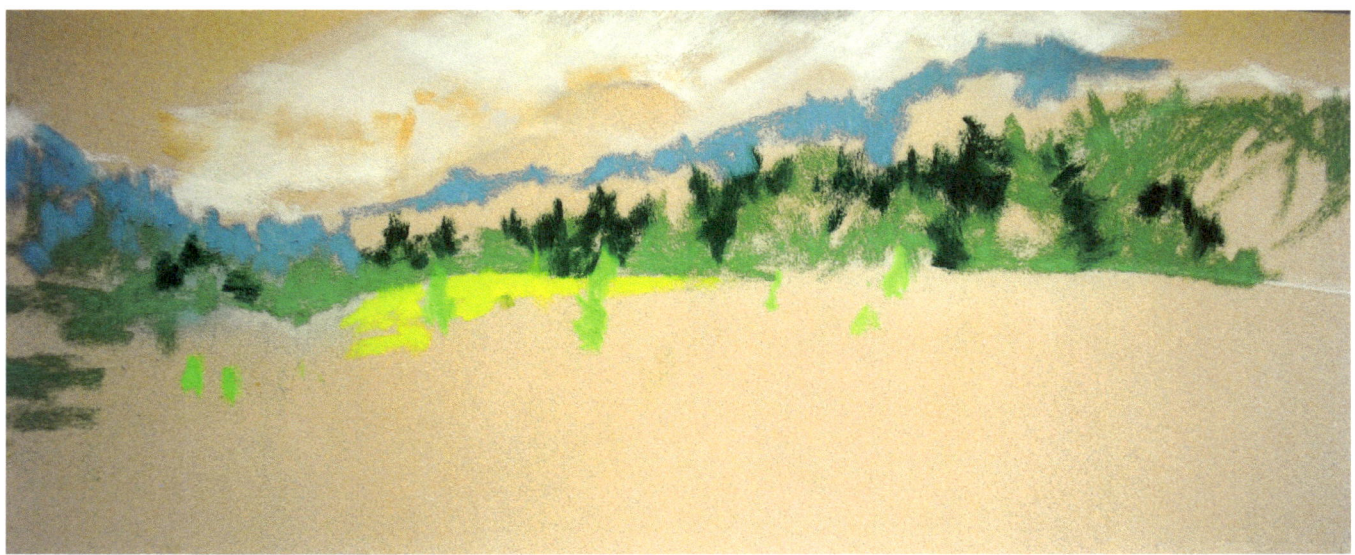

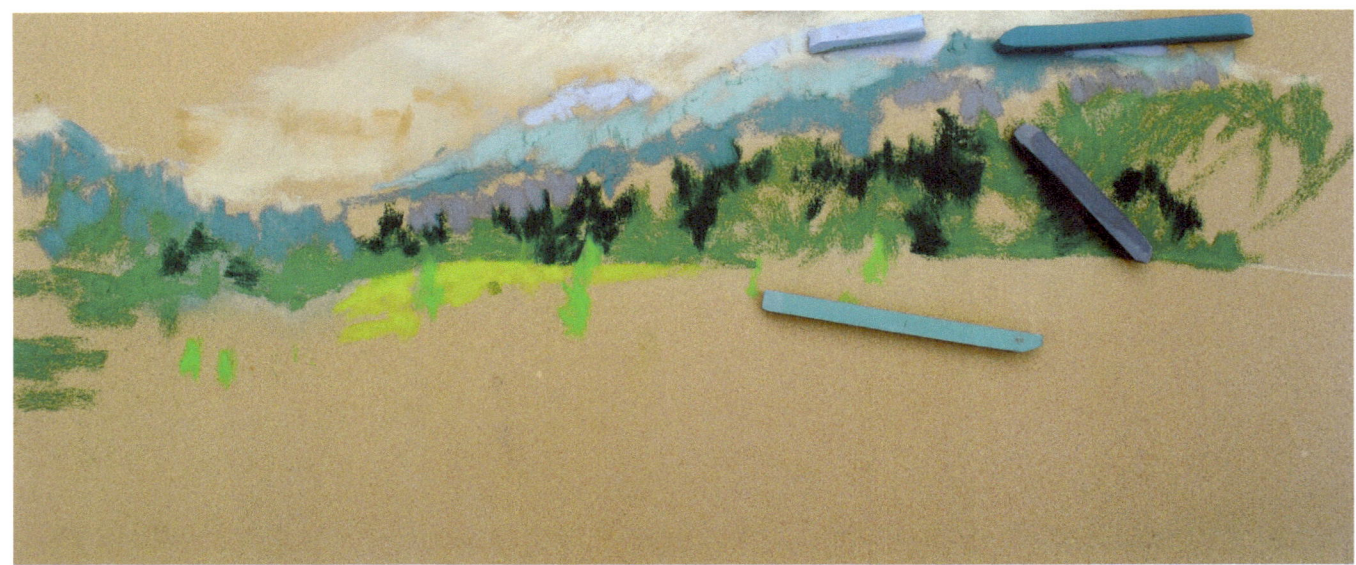

Working on a transition back into the distance, I designate a color for each step back—choosing a sequence related in color—cooler in color and each step back less saturated with color. The early morning light is beautiful but it moves so fast and changes the landscape in front of you dramatically in just a few seconds—it is quite an event! There is no way to keep up with this changing light, but each mark you make with your pastel enhances your sense of sight, sound, smell, and touch to remember the event.

Where there is little light, there is little color and the foreground is still in the shadow of the night. There is a difference between the lack of light at night and an area in shadow from a mountain, tree, or cloud during the day. Sunlight reflects off everything in the daytime, and this reflected light adds interest to the shadows. There is not much color at all at night.

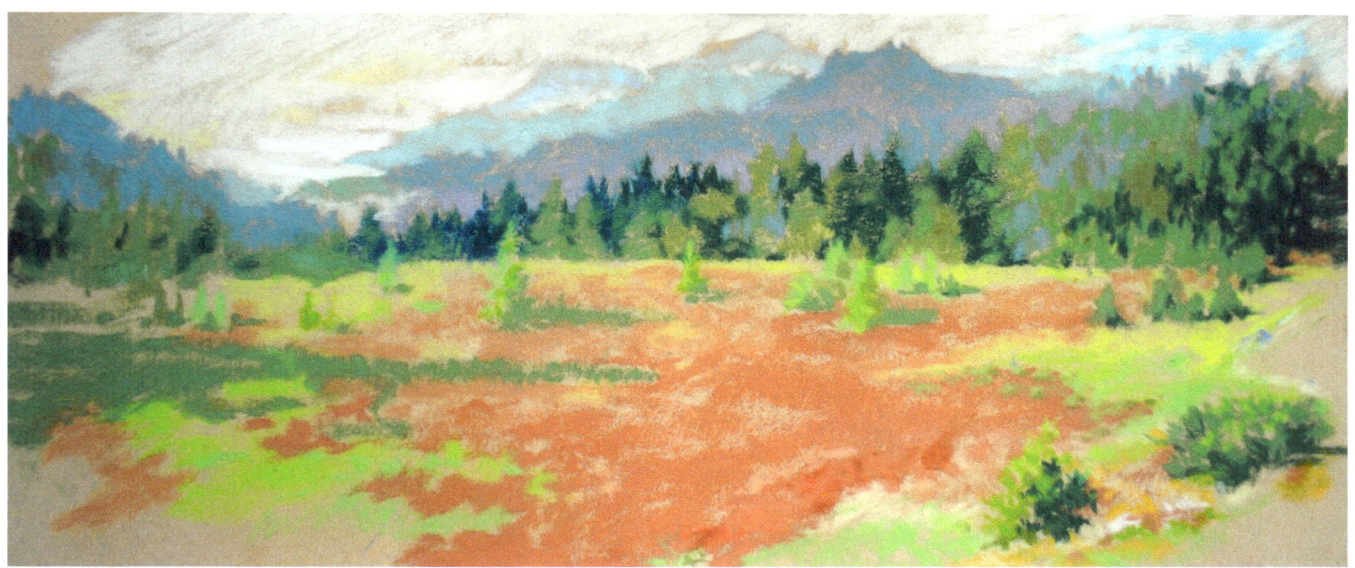

The sun is up! The red earth is a perfect color for making the foreground appear closer. Even though the area where I first started—the back edge of the middle ground—is my focus, the foreground becomes my subject for a short time while I watch the sun stretch across the landscape. I need to keep the red earth on that back edge a cooler red.

You can optically mix pastels by placing two colors next to each other. You can also gray a color by placing its compliment (color on the opposite side of the color wheel) near the color. Green is the compliment of red. I add a few dots of green to keep that back edge cooler and receding.

"There is scarcely any subject that has so many practical and scientific aspects as the subject of color. Its great importance in the arts and the contribution to the enjoyment of life."
—Henry Lefavour

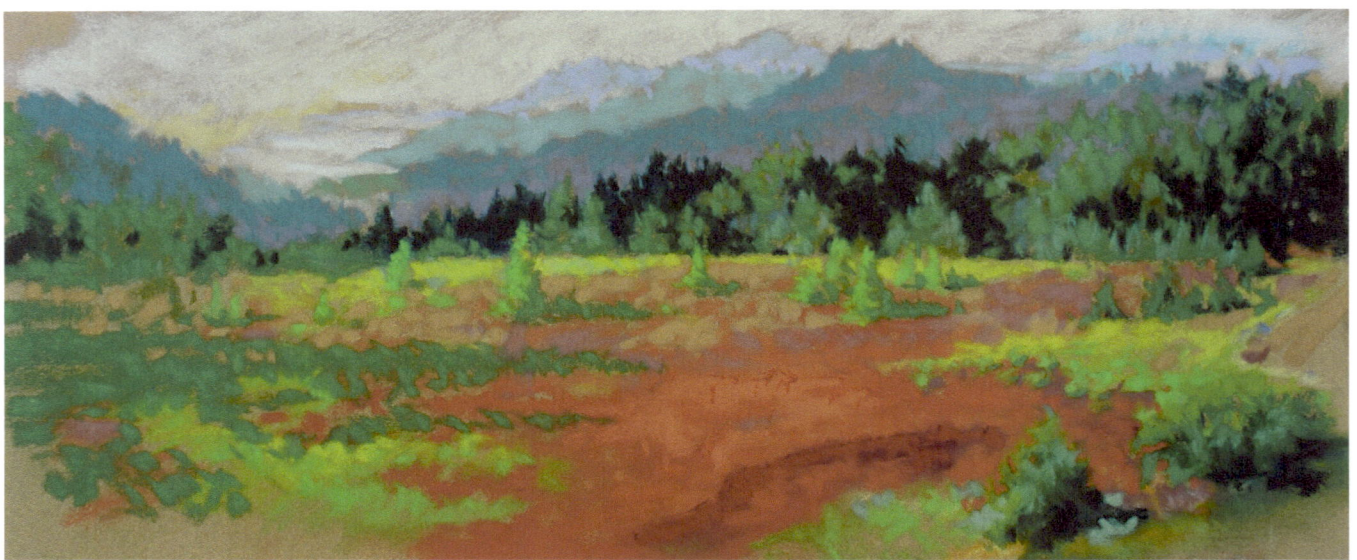

Crater Lake landscape has become the time lapse record of the morning sunrise. Each time I visit the small painting which sits in my studio, I am reminded of such a pleasant place and time. If you take just one hour to draw the landscape, as you travel, you will become connected to this place as never before.

"I believe, above all, that art exists to celebrate, exalt, excite, and satisfy the demands of the visual."
—Wolf Kahn, pastel painter

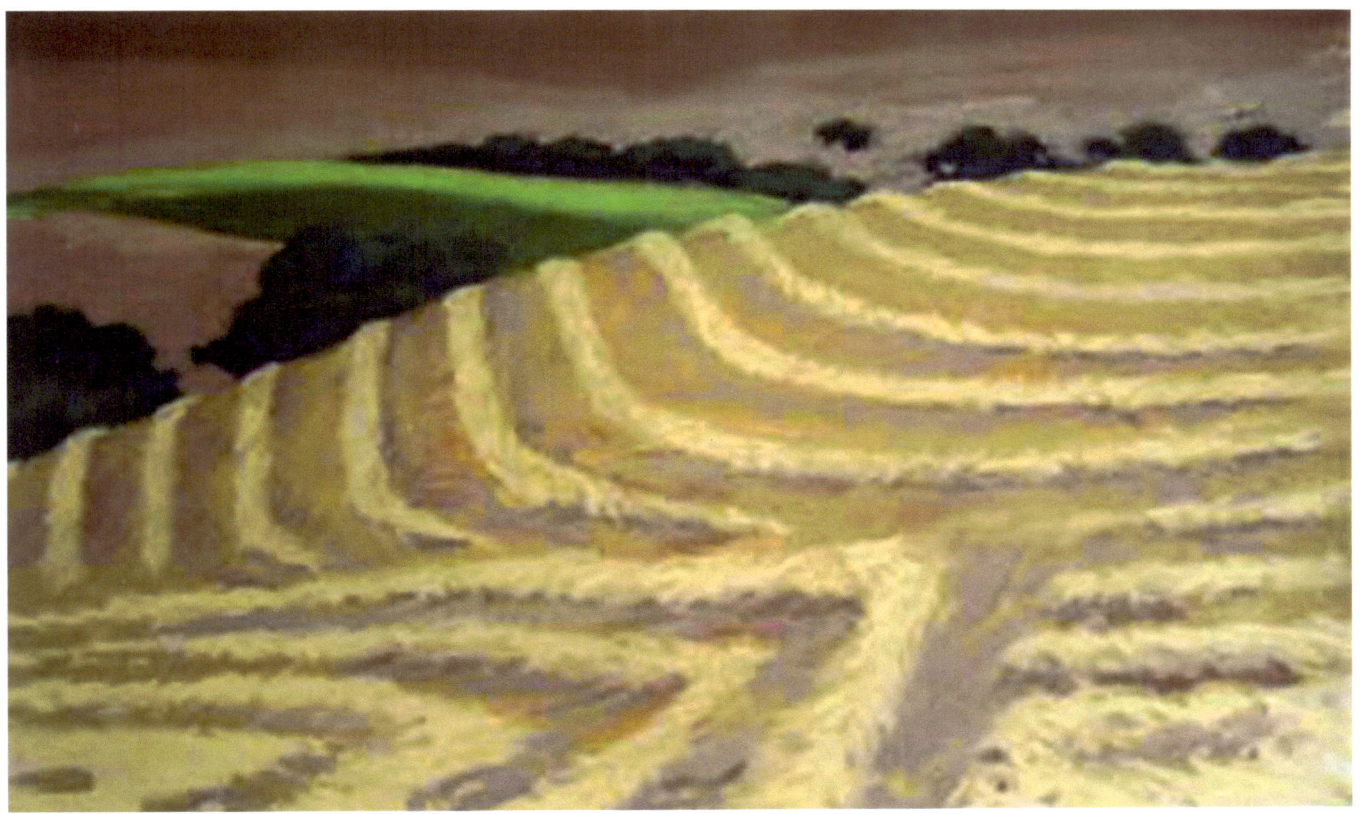

There are many avenues leading to the illusion of deep space—the change in color from warm to cool, the relationship of large objects to smaller objects, a path diminishing in the distance, and even plowed fields. There is inspiration in the ability to express deep space on the flat plane of your drawing surface. It is an educational journey that provides a true sense of accomplishment primarily for the doer. The viewer often takes it for granted, but to the artist, it is magical in a very unique way. I believe we need vistas to gaze upon.

California Field, Pastel on Wallis sanded paper, 10 in. x 18 in.
by Alexia Scott, Summer 2005

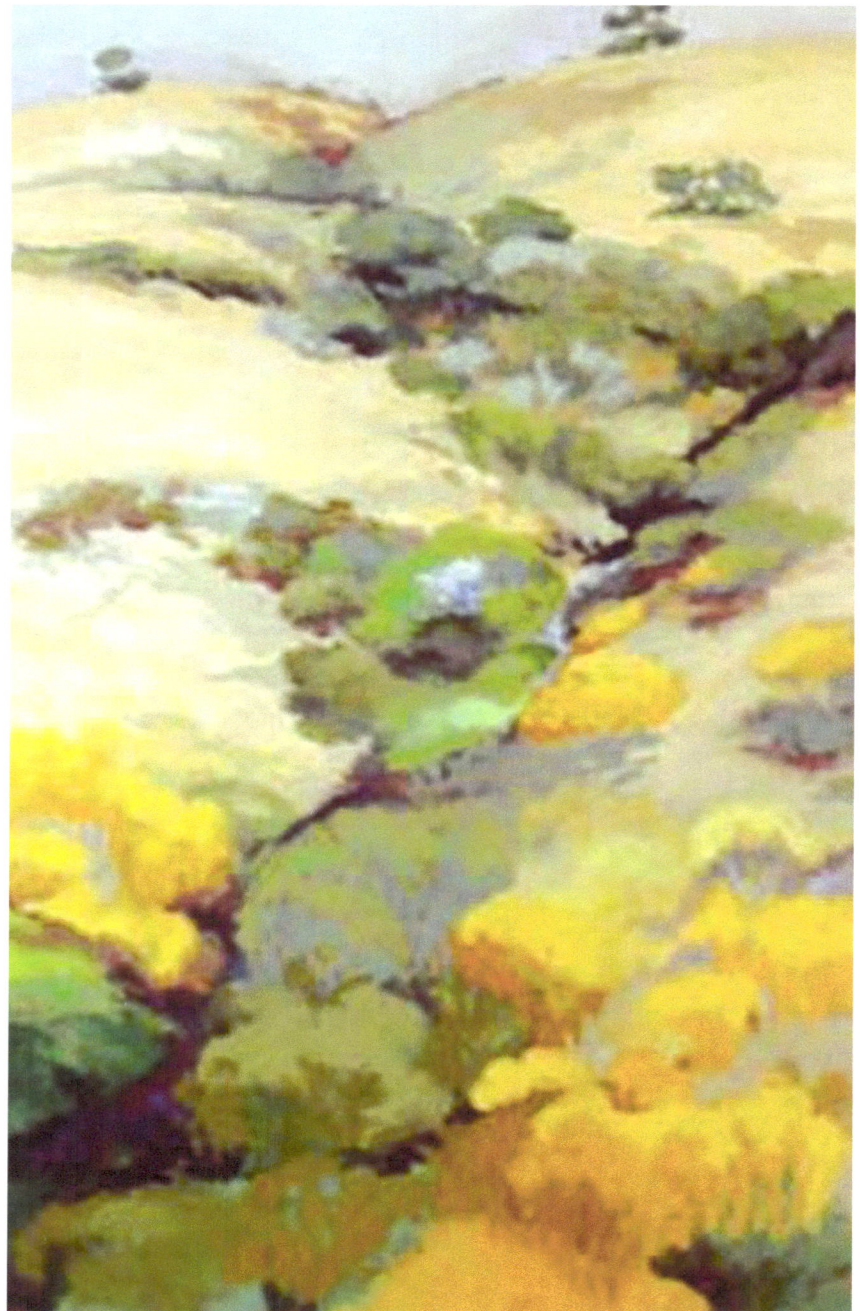

The California hillside, (pictured left), is typical of the smooth rounded hills in the Central Valley. The illusion of deep space is created by changing the size of the trees and foliage from the front larger trees to the small suggestion of trees in the distance. The warm yellow shrubs dominate the foreground, with cooler plants in the back. The valleys are more fertile in this arid climate providing good contrast and welcoming feminine forms.

California Hillside
Pastel on Wallis sanded paper, 24 in. x 34 in.
by Alexia Scott, Summer 2005

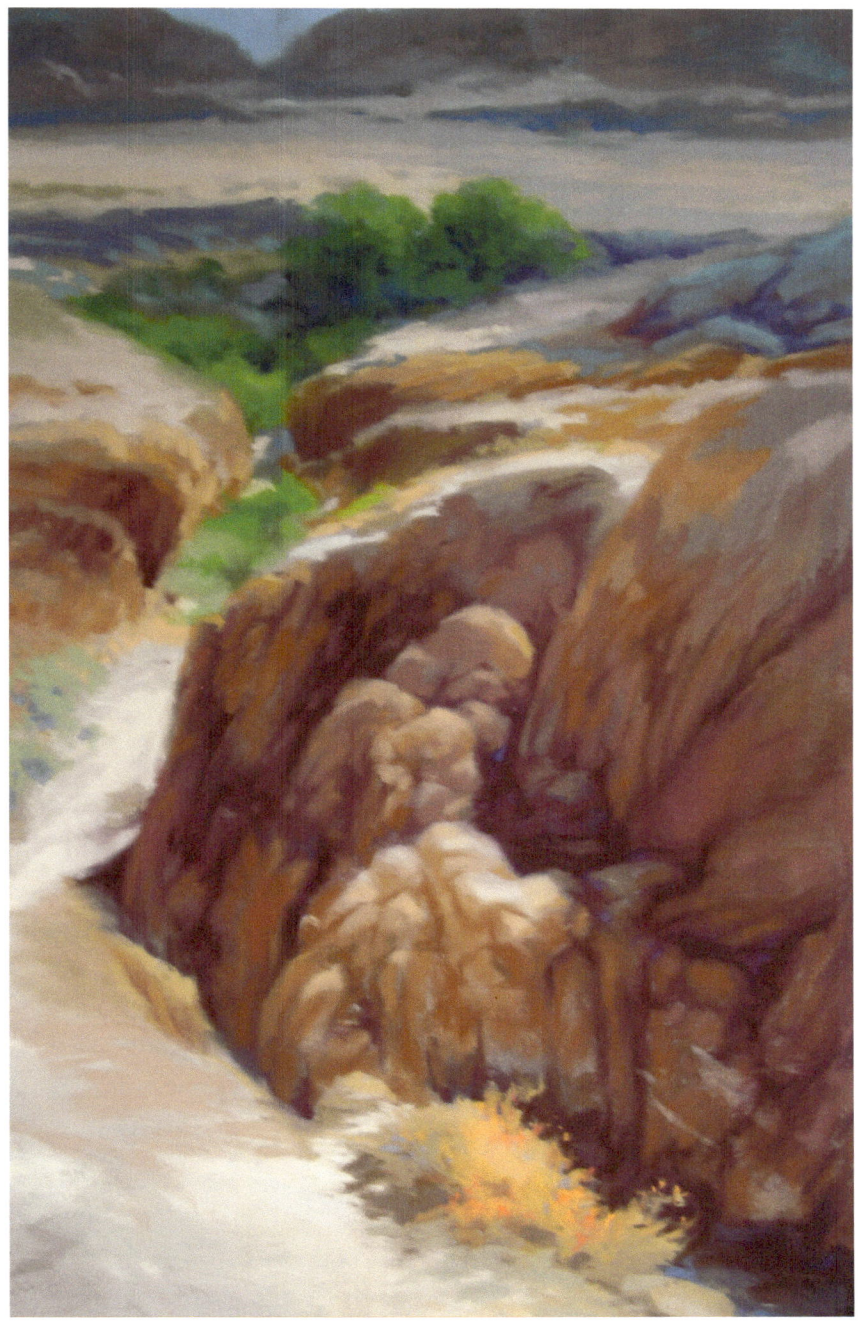

The Alabama Hills outside Lone Pine, CA, are the settings and film locations of several hundred movies from old John Wayne westerns to Star Trek. The red rock hills are an outcropping of red sandstone rock displayed against the gray granite of 14,000 ft. Mt. Whitney and the Sierra Nevada Mountains.

Due to the continued use by the movie industry, the area is left to its natural state. The Dow Hotel will give you a simple map to note many of the film locations. The illusion of deep space (pictured left) is somewhat of a trick used by filmmakers—the warm color and gray background are a perfect composition for distance.

Gunga Din
Pastel, 24 in. x 35 in.
by Alexia Scott, Summer 2005
Location of a bridge from the movie Gunga Din.

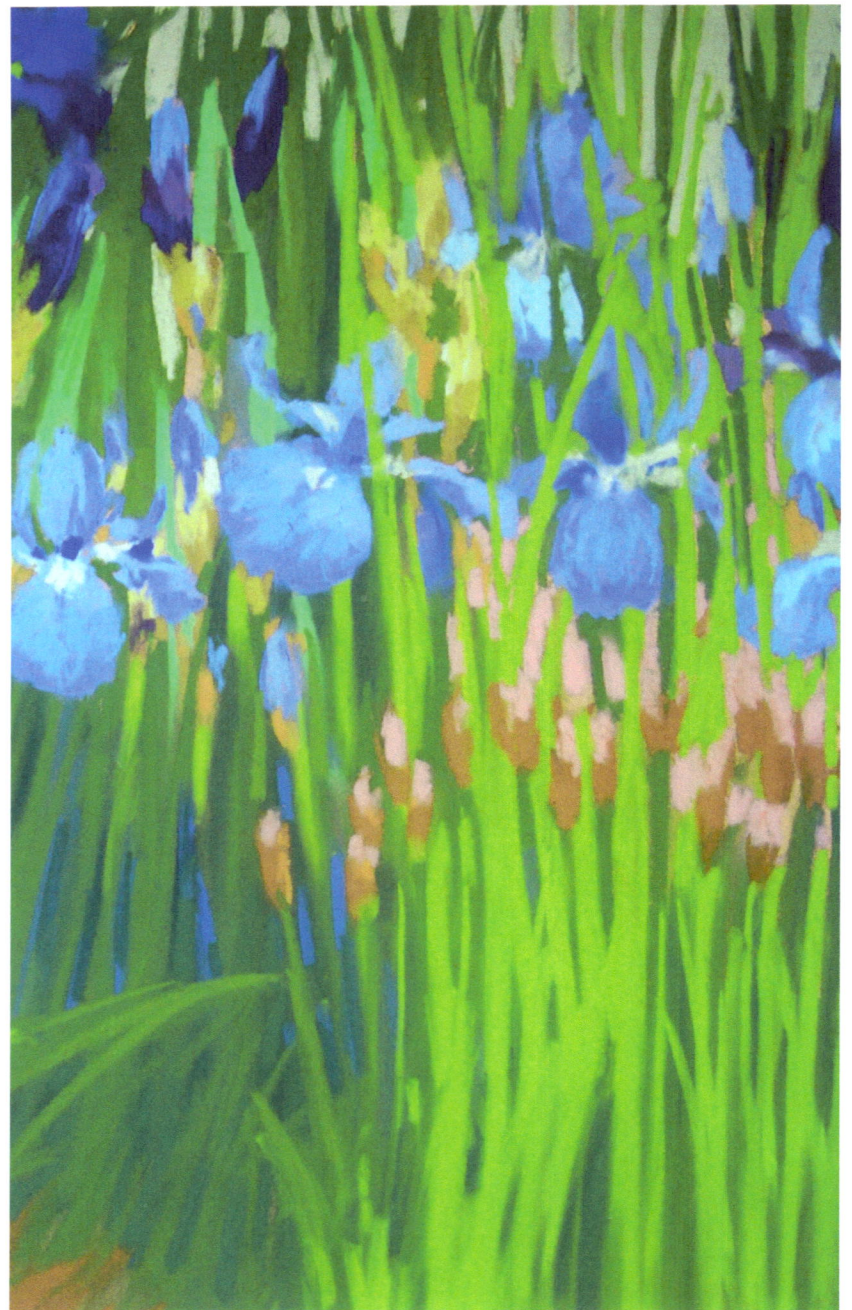

Shallow Space

Working in the garden is relaxing and makes you feel productive. The philosopher Confusious once said that if you want to be happy for the rest of your life, "plant a garden." Painting in the garden is extremely enjoyable and you also gain a sense of accomplishment. The garden does not have to be your own. Most nature centers and public gardens are happy to see artists present and working on location. It adds a different perspective for visitors because they can see the garden through the artist's eyes, as well as their own. Shallow space is kind of an "in your face"—painting, close at hand and filled with complex structures. The overlapping and entwining foliage and the variety of stems and flowers will create complex abstract forms within the picture plane frame.

Anne's Iris - detail
Pastel on Wallis sanded paper.
by Alexia Scott, May 2010,
Painted in a friend's garden in Great Falls, VA

It is well documented that the receding space in landscapes provides a restful view; however, the complexities of the "in your face" garden composition is especially engaging while working with your subject. All external thoughts become relegated to the dusty corners of your left brain while the painting is in process.

The interesting compositions that look so complicated can be achieved by beginning with the structures closest to you and working your way back into the shallow space. All the while, looking for the filtering light prancing around the stems and leaves. A leaf is rarely all the same color of green unless it is deep in the plant with no light. That being said, compositionally, you will need some quieter areas. Do not allow the background to just be a background color. Draw your background by drawing the negative space between your structures.

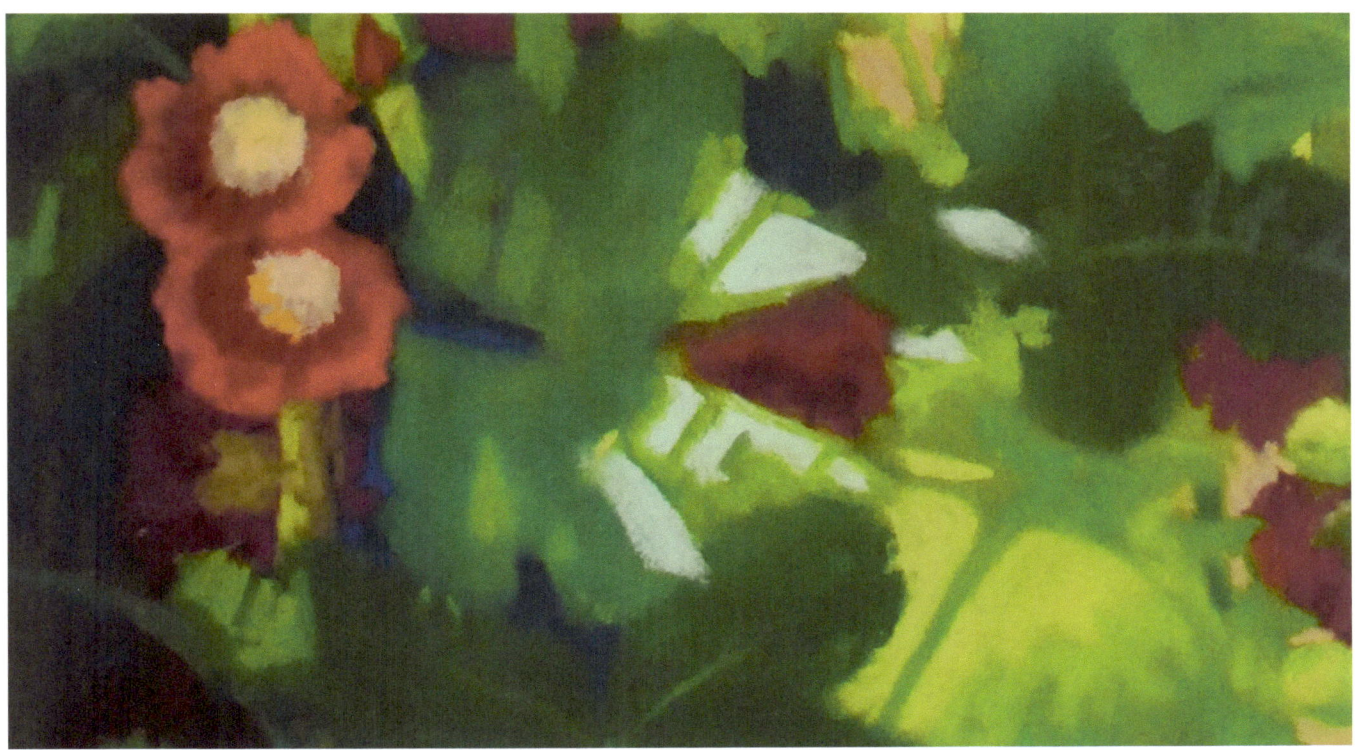

Color Is Relative, Pastel, 20 in. x 24 in.
by Alexia Scott

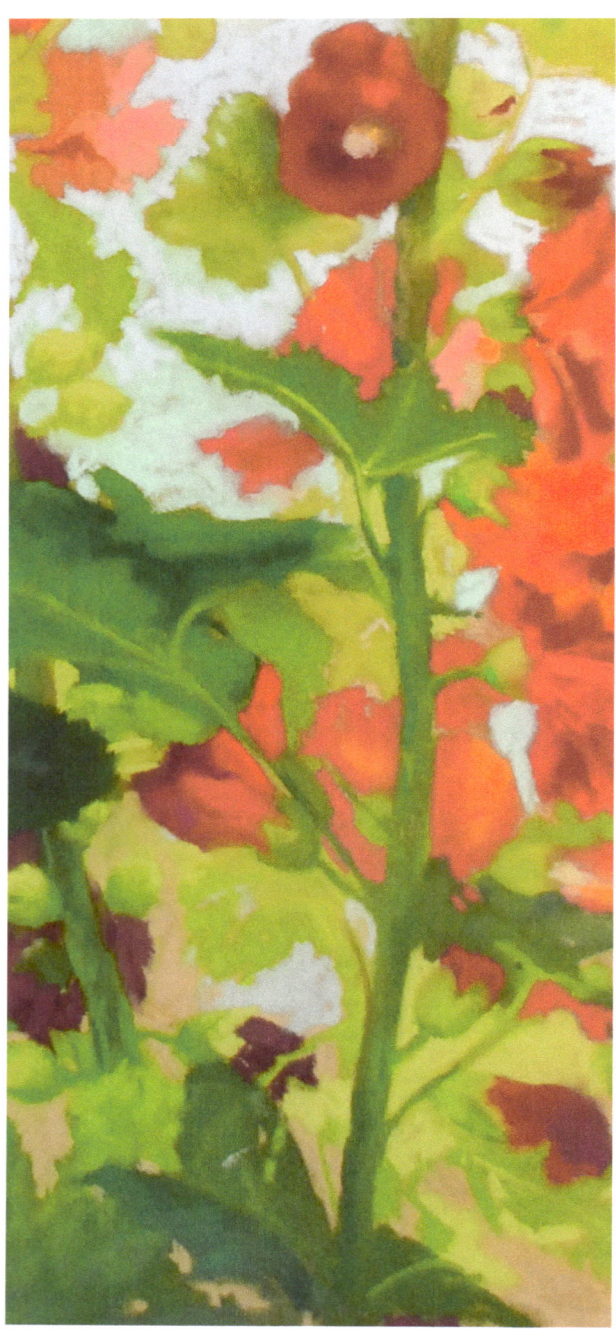

This negative space is as important as the positive space, or your subject, because your sight registers the negative space while determining what you are looking at. The brain registers edges and shapes before detail, and you should too.

These detail selections show an area in the composition where the sunlight is hitting on part of a leaf and also creating a shadow from another part of the plant structure on a leaf. Notice the contrast and calming effect of the plain leaves toward the bottom of the plant. The detail to the left began with the stem, leaf, and flower in the foreground, and I continued to work back into the space.

There is so much information at hand in the garden. You can pick and choose what you want. Your painting is your composition and a suggestion of the garden before you. While you work, the light and the wind will constantly rearrange your subject, but as you draw, you will understand the plant's personality and paint it as you would a friend.

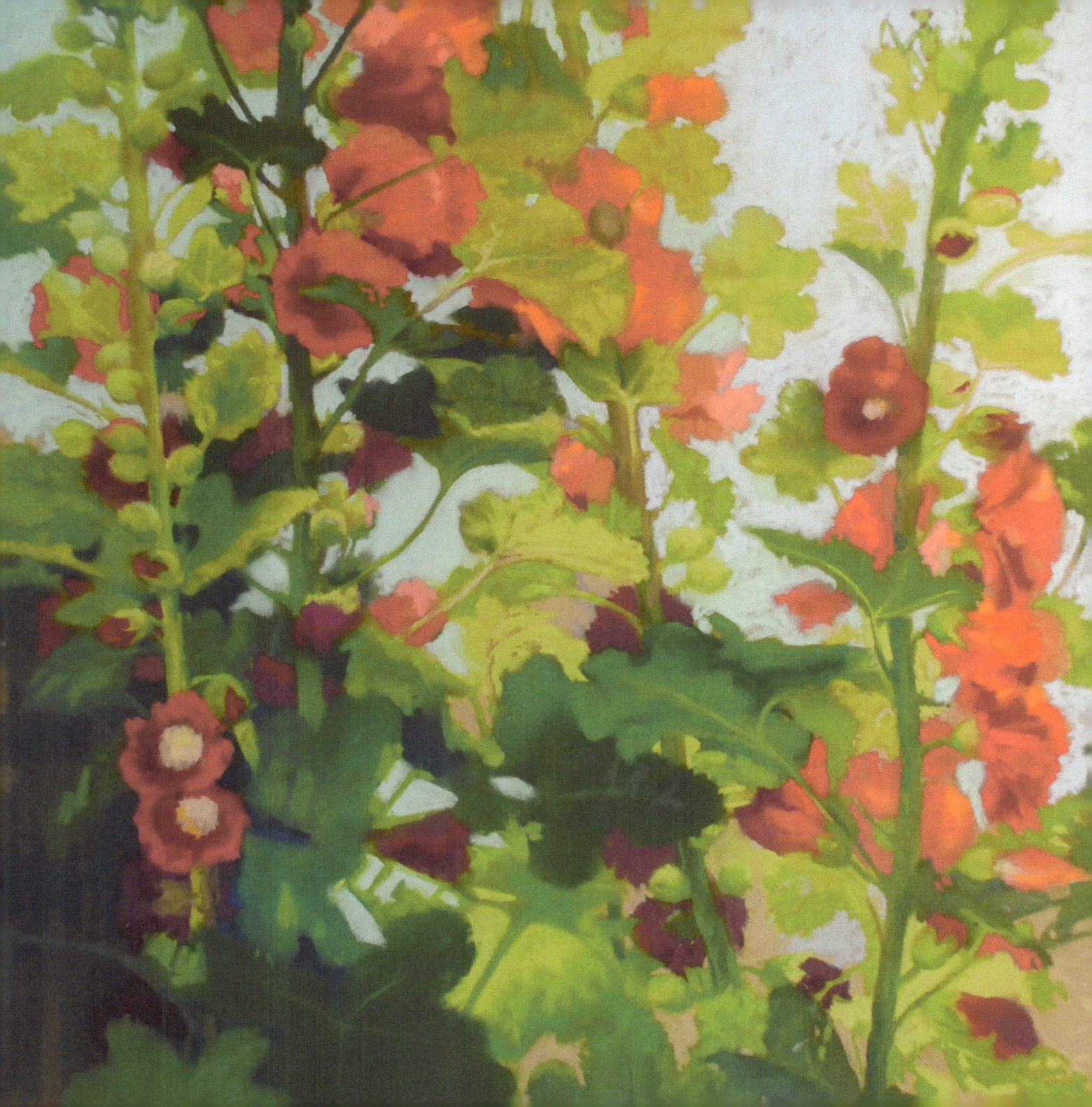

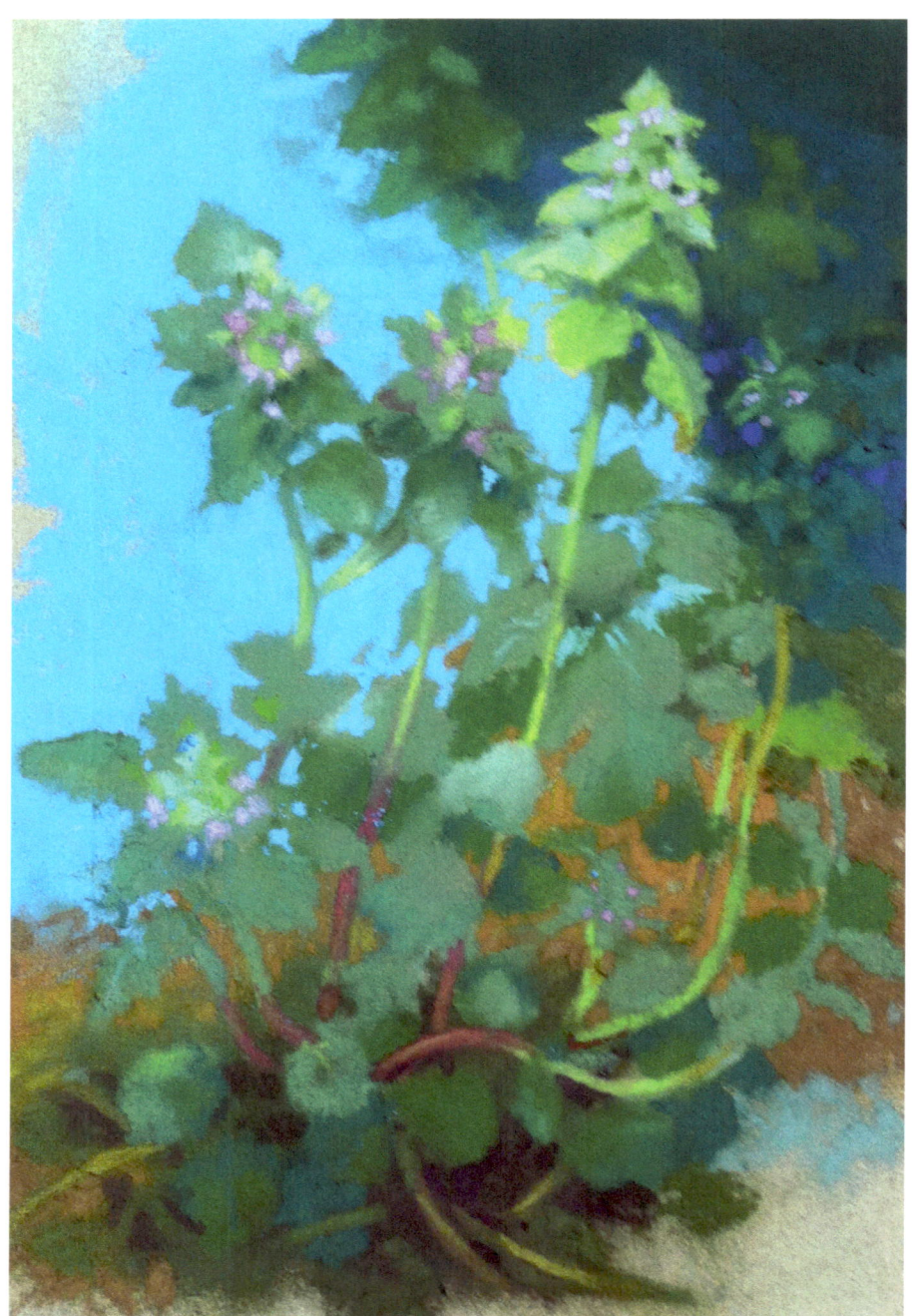

The Weed in My Walk
Pastel on La Carte paper, 8 in. x 10 in.
by Alexia Scott, June 2013

I needed to do some weeding, but this is a difficult task when you think everything that grows is interesting. For these small studies, you need to stick with the square pastels as your aim is better in such a tight composition. These weeds just grow by the bunches in my yard. It is time well spent to just sit and draw whatever is there.

Adding Design Principles—Unity and Harmony

Painting in the field provides you with a huge amount of visual information which needs to be edited and controlled. I often find it useful to do a pastel painting of an area before I do a large oil painting. The pastels are a doodling tool that can help you find your way through a tangled mess, because everything can be easily reconfigured to suit your purpose. The idea of a painting having a purpose is something to remember. Just like an essay has a story to tell, so does a painting. Rambling on about this or that in an essay does not make it a good essay—and it is the same in landscape painting. Pick a focus, decide why you want to paint this scene, and keep this in mind while you are working. You will need to edit what you see and minimize the areas that draw attention away from the focus.

The pastel *Red with Greens* (pictured right) began with the arching stems and lime green color. All of the principles of design overlap in theory. Unity and harmony are design principles that focus on placement. Is there any element of the composition that is out of character? The wrong color or placement can annoy the viewer and/or the artist.

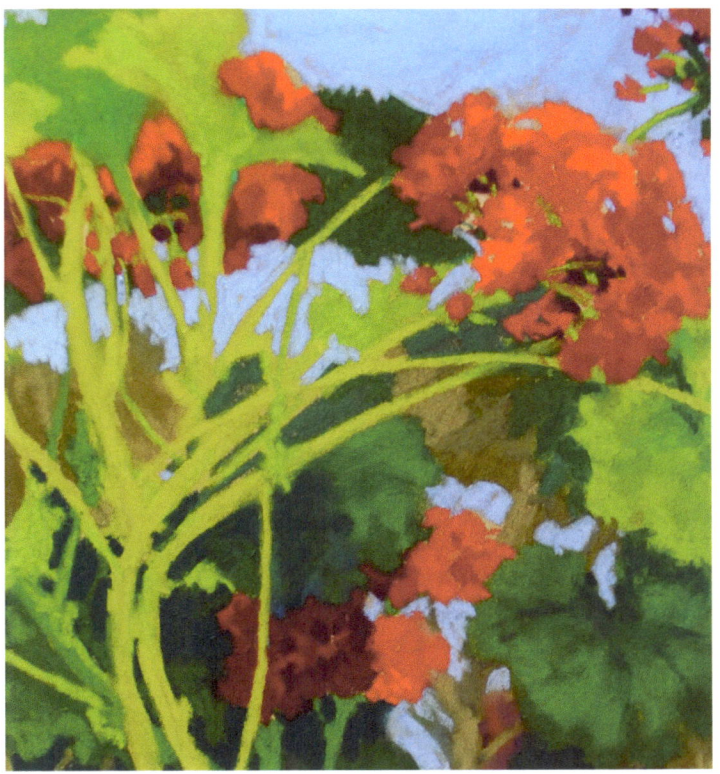

Composition is another aspect of a natural understanding of visual language. It is hard to teach, but it is something most people know. You will hear people say "well I know what I like." Trained artists tend to dismiss this idea, but, in fact, there is some truth to it. The problem is they cannot explain why they know what they like and this is what you can learn through an understanding of design.

Balance

Balance is another form of unity. It is the equilibrium in the painting that creates a feeling of calmness. In some artwork, you may deliberately create an unbalanced structure. Here we are illustrating calmness. The detail (pictured below) is an area of quiet structures to balance the reaching bright green stems of the painting. In the English language, we read from left to right; this also has an effect on the balance of the painting. I placed my most active structure at the first place we look and subordinated the rest of the picture to this area. However, as you explore the shallow layers, you can find passages of secondary interest.

Rhythm and Repetition

Rhythm and repetition seem to go hand-in-hand while creating a composition, because the rhythm is often suggested by repetition of color and/or form. The pastel marks and brush strokes can suggest rhythm. Here, the rhythm is red. It is important to understand the emotional link humans have to rhythm and repetition—we are comforted by it. In music, rhythm and repetition are soothing elements and, in painting, we respond to them the same way.

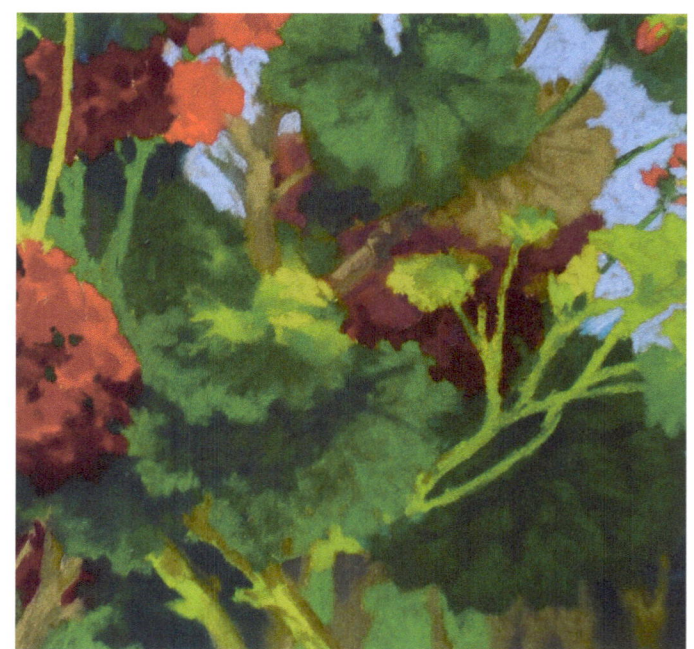

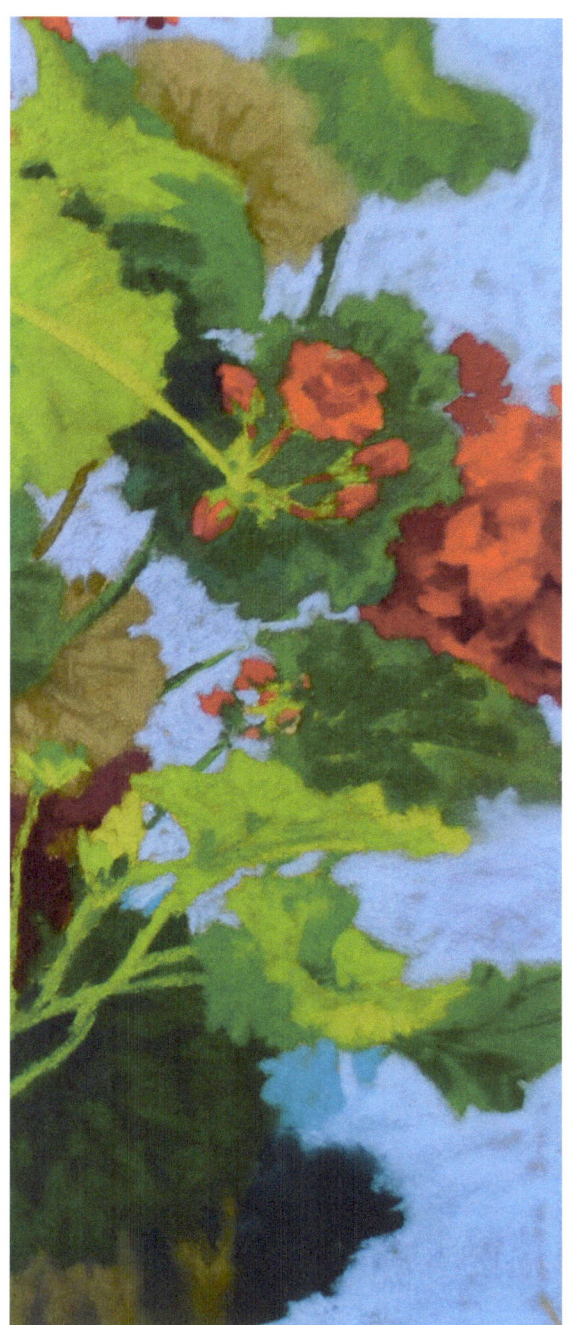

Colors on a canvas are like musical notes creating a visual composition. Placement of the musical notes and the visual elements are important and create unity within the picture plane. The more we understand our natural visual language, the better we understand what elements in our field studies will grant us the most inner fulfillment. The detail (pictured left) suggests variations on a theme to move the eye around the painting. The areas reaching off the edges places the viewer in the garden with more garden beyond.

Symmetry and Asymmetry

Symmetry and asymmetry are two types of balance. Symmetry is generally formal—placing the flowers in the middle of a table. Asymmetry is informal—placing flowers to the side of center and a book near them to balance the space. *Red with Greens* is clearly an example of asymmetry.

Next page: *Red with Greens*, Pastel on La Carte Pastel Card in antique white, 15 in. x 15 in.
by Alexia Scott, July 2013
This is the full size image of the pastel. I was painting on my patio in Falls Church, VA, and because I was close to my studio I selected additional green pastels for my composition.

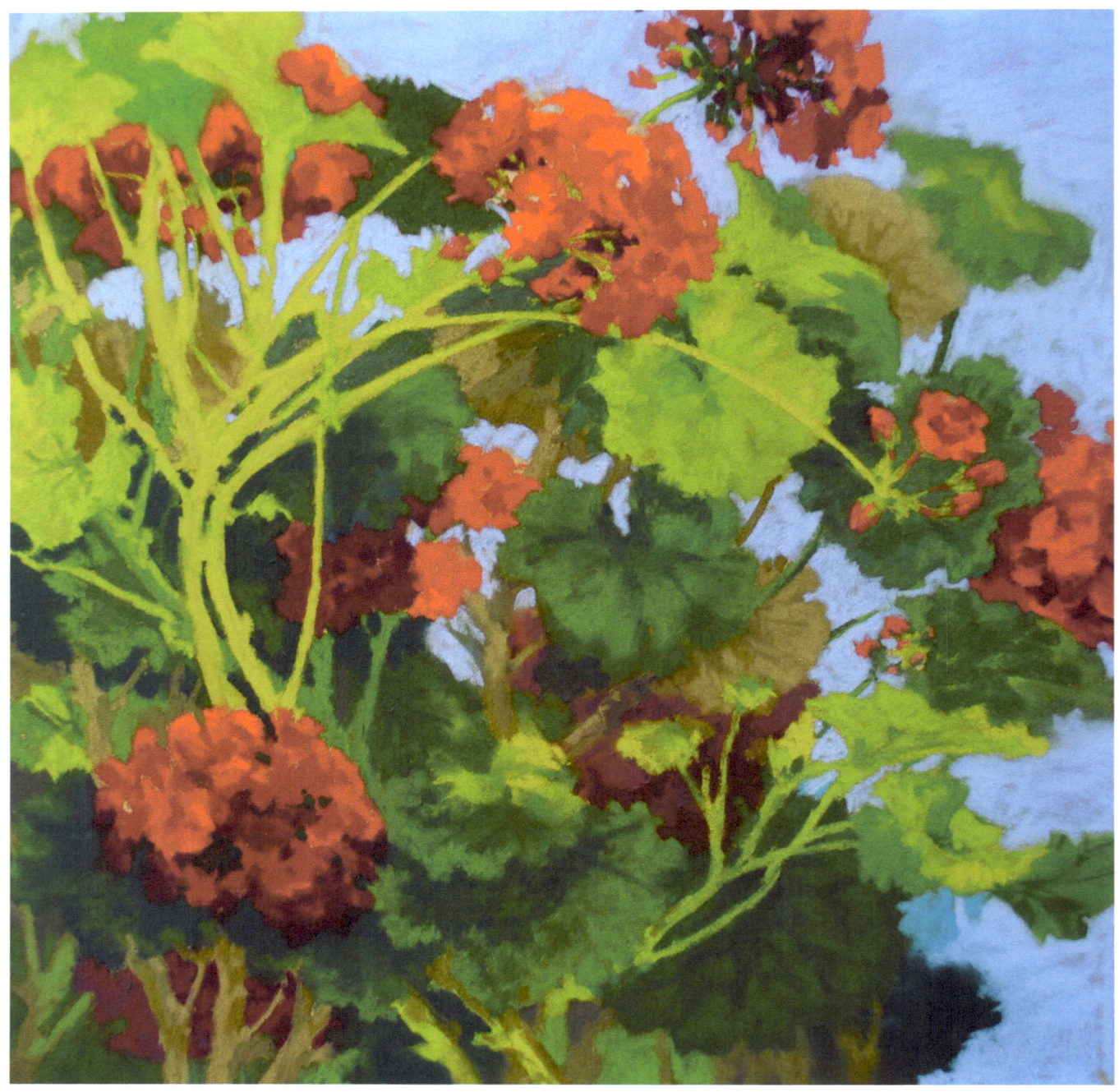

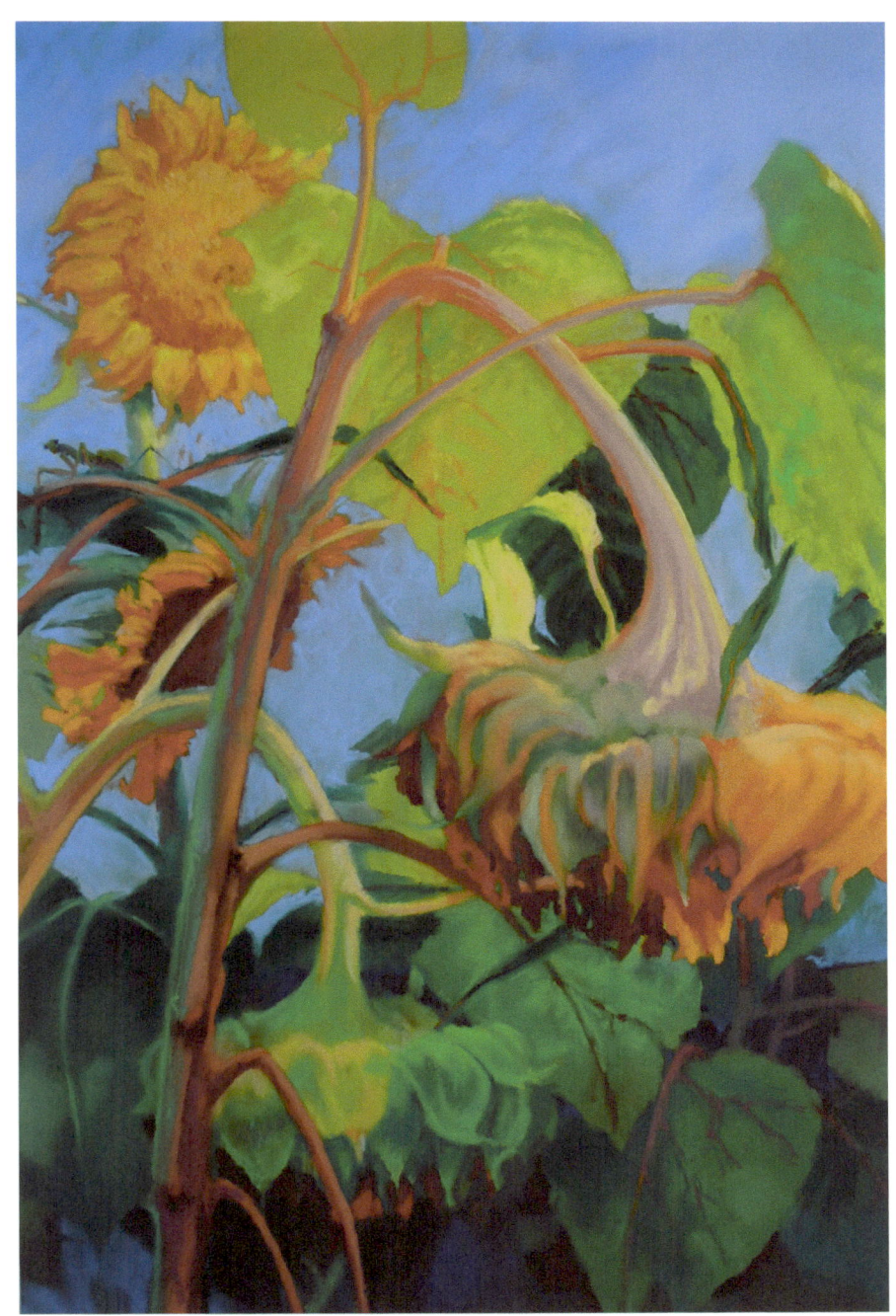

When Sunflower are Young They Follow The Sun, Pastel on La Carte Pastel Card by Alexia Scott

Each summer, I plant sunflowers just to paint them. I began this painting with the large flower bent over by the maturing seeds. From this study, I continued back into the sunflower patch selecting the individuals I wanted for the composition. This shallow space study provides visual elements for exploration and a home for the mantis in the upper left of the garden.

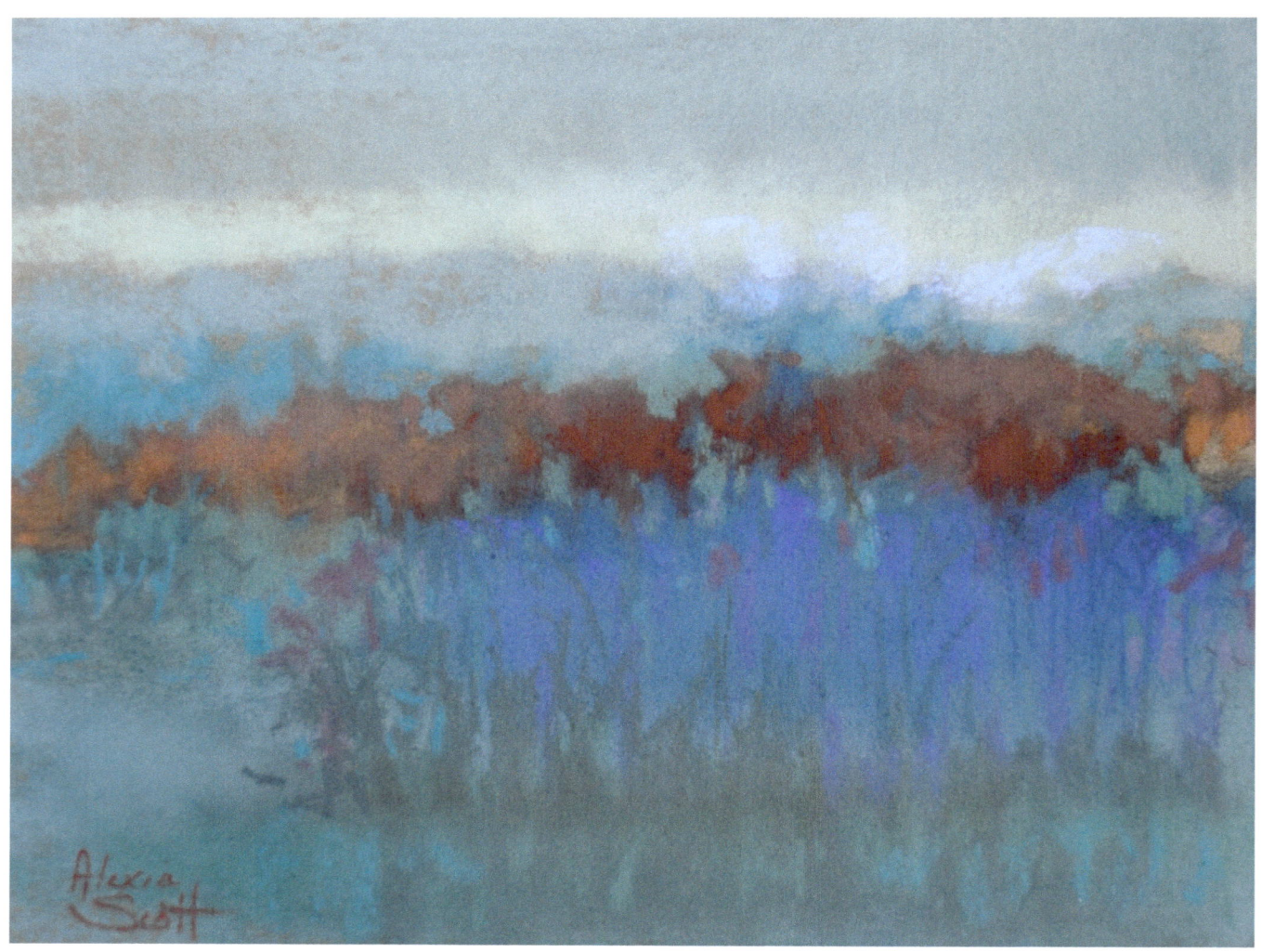

Potomac Fog Study, Pastel, 7 in. x 9 in.
by Alexia Scott, October 2009

Looking across the river from my third floor window in the Torpedo Factory Art Center, Alexandria, VA, the fog created subtle colors with the emerging fall foliage.

Fog is Fun

A good way to understand the concept of space is to spend some time drawing the landscape on a foggy or rainy day. At this time, the atmospheric perspective is exaggerated. This changes the color and value as you recede in space. The filtering light creates unusual reflected colors, and cooler colors seem to pop a little.

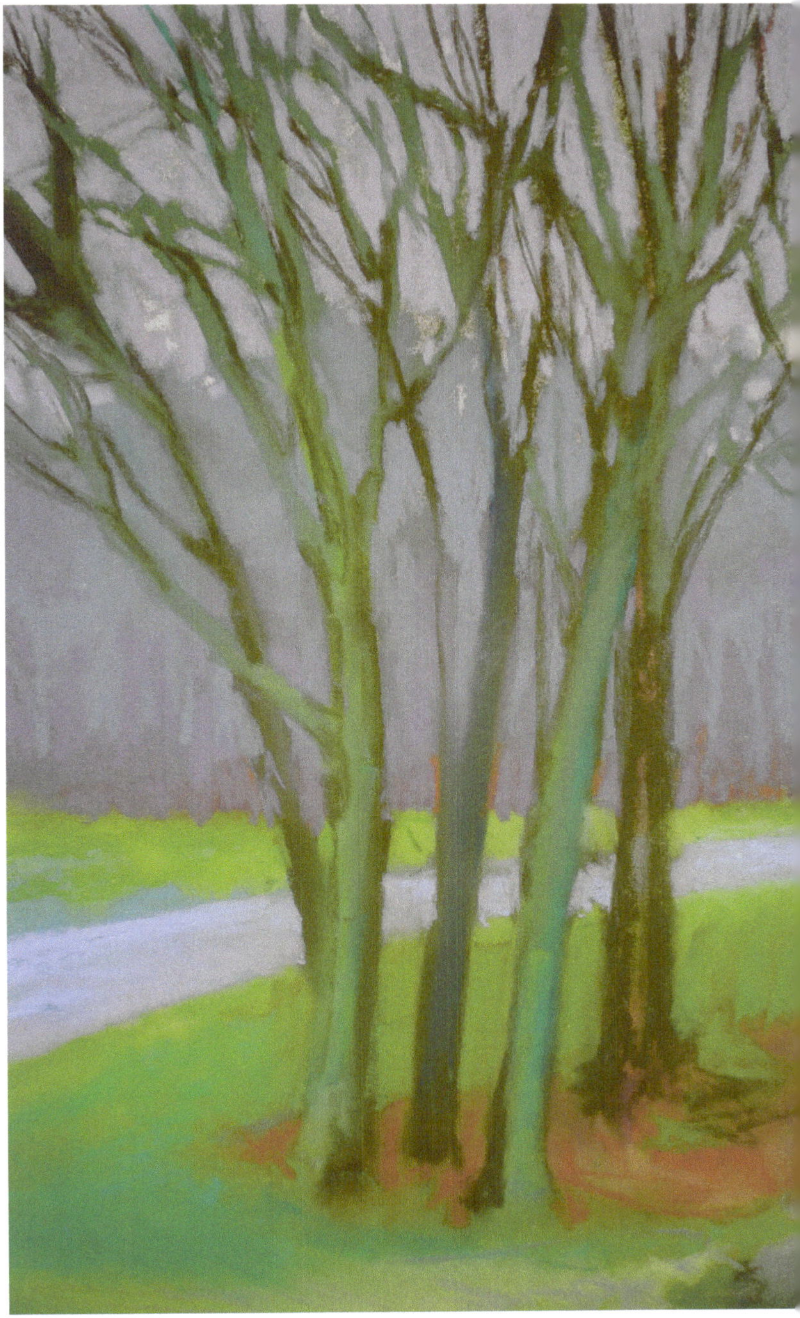

Green Trees, Pastel, 12 in. x 9 in.
by Alexia Scott, November 2010

Painted near the lodge at Big Meadows, Shenandoah National Park, VA, this small study was inspired by green. The moss on the trees and the fog seemed to make the green stand out in an unusual way. I was sitting in the parking lot with my [always present] pastel bag and did a quick study. Keeping your equipment simple is important.

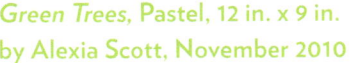

Study or Painting

I should clarify the difference between a study and a painting. All paintings are studies, but they also incorporate the added elements of design, composition, attention to the picture plane edges, and everything discussed so far. The study is just that. You will study one thing and the end result will be knowledge, but not necessarily a good painting. Sometimes they are wonderful, but it is not the end goal. In all artistic endeavors, you should be willing to make a mess, make mistakes, and work only for the sake of learning. There are no shortcuts in art, but there are shortcuts to a feeling of enjoyment and time spent with nature.

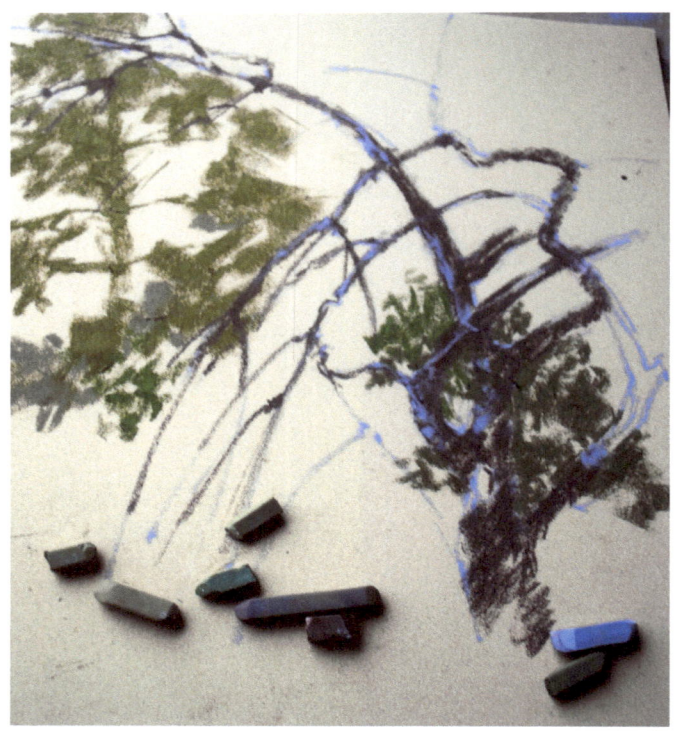

The study is your key, no pressure. Just put the picture in a folder when you finish. The knowledge you have gained has added to your visual vocabulary and will enhance your next study. At Georgetown University, my athletic students, in particular, understood the importance of practice. Many people have the mistaken idea that art is different than other skills and is not something you can learn. This is not the case, however, and practice is a great teacher.

Right Image: *The Fog Study,* La Carte Pastel Card
by Alexia Scott, January 2014
Falls Church, VA studio window. At this point, you will need the additional box of Prismacolor Nupastels. They contain a nice selection of warm and cool grays. Grays and natural colors do not look very exciting, but learning how to use them will greatly enhance your work.

January 2014 has only given us 11 days to date, yet we have had 4 inches of snow, 3 days at 5 to 11 degrees, rain, and fog—a weatherman's dream and great fun for nature studies. There is nothing better during these days than to sit at a window and draw whatever we can see. Certainly not as grand as summer studies, but beneficial in their own right. The connection with nature and the learning that will follow is good for your mental health and artistic skills. When I work in low light or limited values, I look for whatever color I can find and give it a little tweak. There are the grays which could dominate the day, but if you find closely related colors, mix them in or make them up.

Since the sky is overcast, the sun will not shine on any part of the subject so the depiction of volume is flattened out. The darker tree in the foreground is more of a design than a tree, with volume and mass. It is almost difficult to see where the branches overlap as the values are so closely related. The volume of any object is recognized by light

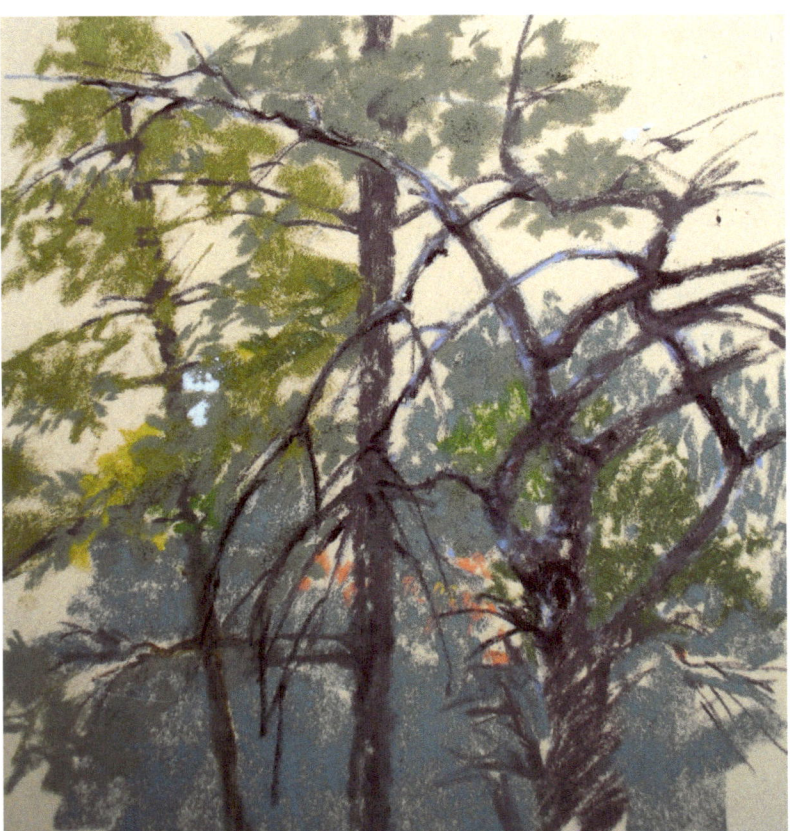

hitting on a portion of the surface—no light equals no volume, but there is still structure. When you collect the pastels you want to use, keep them separate from the rest. Sometimes I use a small, flat lid to place the pastels I am using in. Now that you are using more pastels, you would be surprised how difficult it is to know which ones you are using if they get mixed together. Notice the light blue dots in the middle left? They are the wrong color, and it is obvious.

I photographed the first two demos on my lap in the foggy light, but for the final one, I photographed it in the sunlight on the next day—interesting difference.

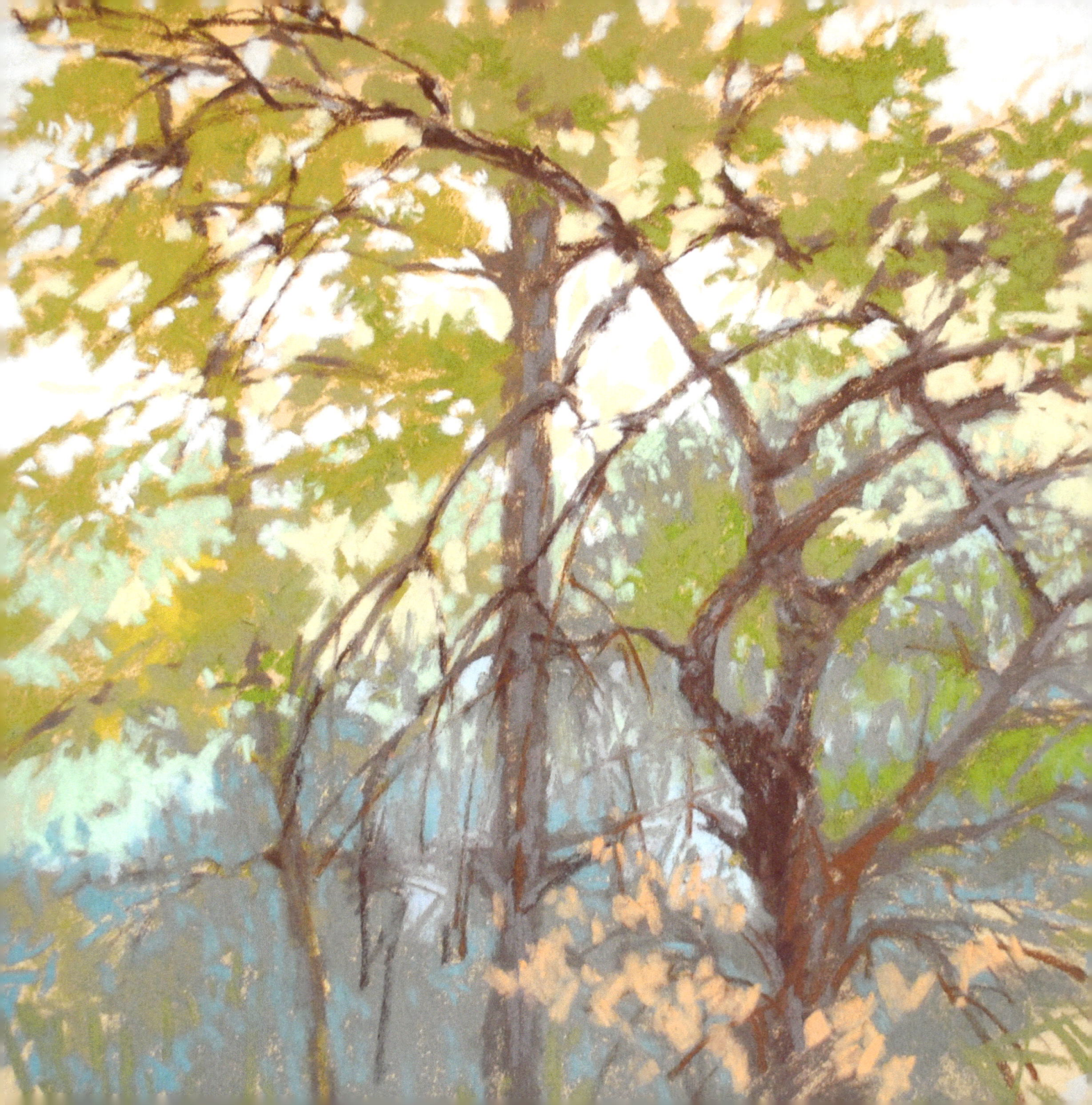

Light Is Your Key

Understand your light: the direction, time of day, full light, defused light, reflected light, and shadowed by a cloud is important. Colors are warmer in the afternoon and cooler in the morning light. The light falling on a tree, hill, or cloud defines the object's shape. While you are working out in the field, pay close attention to the light and its effect on your subject. When you concentrate on your view, analyze what you are seeing. You will be editing the visual information, so it is important to know what to focus on to make the statement you want to make. You can also use these elements to create a better composition. We all paint light. Without light, there is nothing to paint and no color. Even the darkest nocturne has subtle light. Do not take the light for granted. Contemplate its effects on the time and place you are painting.

A FEW COLOR DEFINITIONS

Hue: The term "hue" is the name for a color and its cousins. Blue is a color and all other colors that are blue with a little of this or that, such as greenish blue or blue violet, are referred to as a blue hue.

Value: Dark to light in black and white and in color refers to the color's value. Dark red, medium red, light red are all different values of the same hue.

Intensity: This refers to the purity and brightness of the hue. As you look at your pastels, pick out the brightest ones. These are considered to be the highest in intensity. Dull colors are the lowest in intensity. Some use the term vivid to describe the intensity of a color.

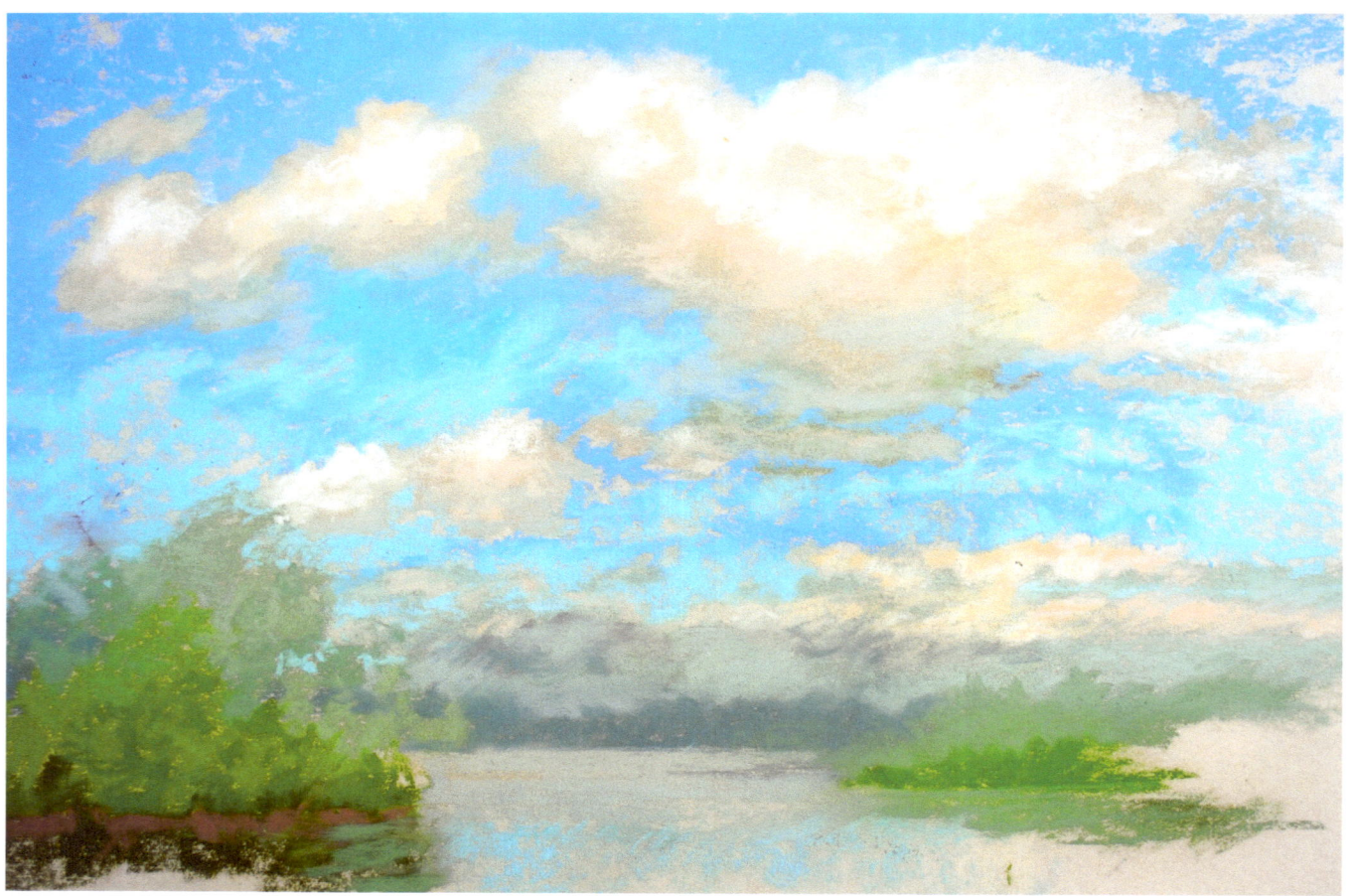

Clouds Keep Moving

It is difficult to find a vista where I live, with so many trees. This cloud study was done in July 2013 on UArt sanded paper (off-white), while I was sitting on a dock on the Occoquan River. Understanding the form and volume of clouds will help you paint them even when the sky is changing rapidly in front of you. Clouds are actually heavy, with great structure that the light shines on while shadows are cast on the ground; really no different than a big, round tree. However, there are many forms of clouds from solid to wispy. Everyone enjoys clouds, and you will enjoy painting them.

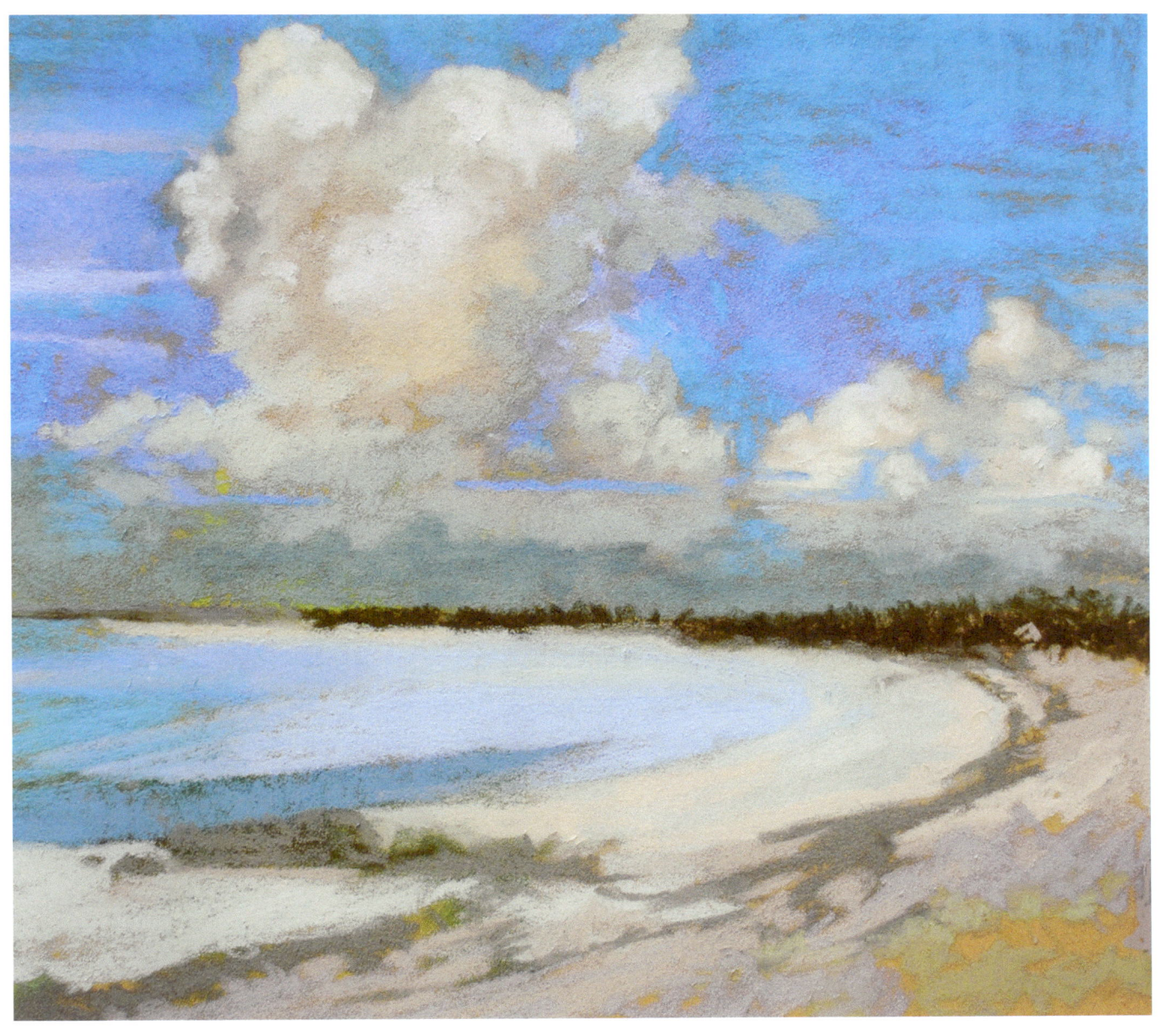

Green Turtle Clouds, Pastel on La Carte Pastel Card, antique white, 10 in. x 10 in.
by Alexia Scott

Clouds are made of water vapor which creates the wispy collections of droplets that are at an altitude where the dew point turns the vapor into droplets. These droplets form into all the different cloud structures, depending on the atmospheric conditions. For our purpose, we need to think about the cloud as both vapor and solid—water and ice. It is very cold aloft and ice crystals form adding color when the sun reflects off the ice and vapors. The cloud has mass and looks white, but it is many colors. The whitest area is where the sun directly hits the surface of the water vapor, the darkest area is away from the light. The closer the water molecules are together, the less light can enter the cloud and reflect back to your eye. It is important to keep the structures of the cloud as an abstract object unit. As you are drawing, the cloud is moving, transforming, merging, and dissipating. If you create a quick gesture drawing of the cloud form, you can use the changing clouds as reference to build the cloud you sketched.

Start With One Cloud

As clouds overlap and become a cluster of clouds, keeping your place as they change is tricky. It is best to draw one cloud and begin to think of them as individuals, not a big mass. This will help you maintain a convincing structure. There is a lot of freedom in landscape painting but understanding the basics will help you be in control of your painting, not the painting in control of you.

CLOUD STUDY

Begin with a quick gesture drawing of the clouds. This will provide you with a framework. You should freeze the cloud in time with the drawing, because it will continue to evolve before you. It is not necessary to be neat with this drawing, as it will be covered up while you work your way through your study. The more gestural you are, the more the volume and mass of the clouds will emerge. I find the La Carte antique white is a good choice for cloud studies.

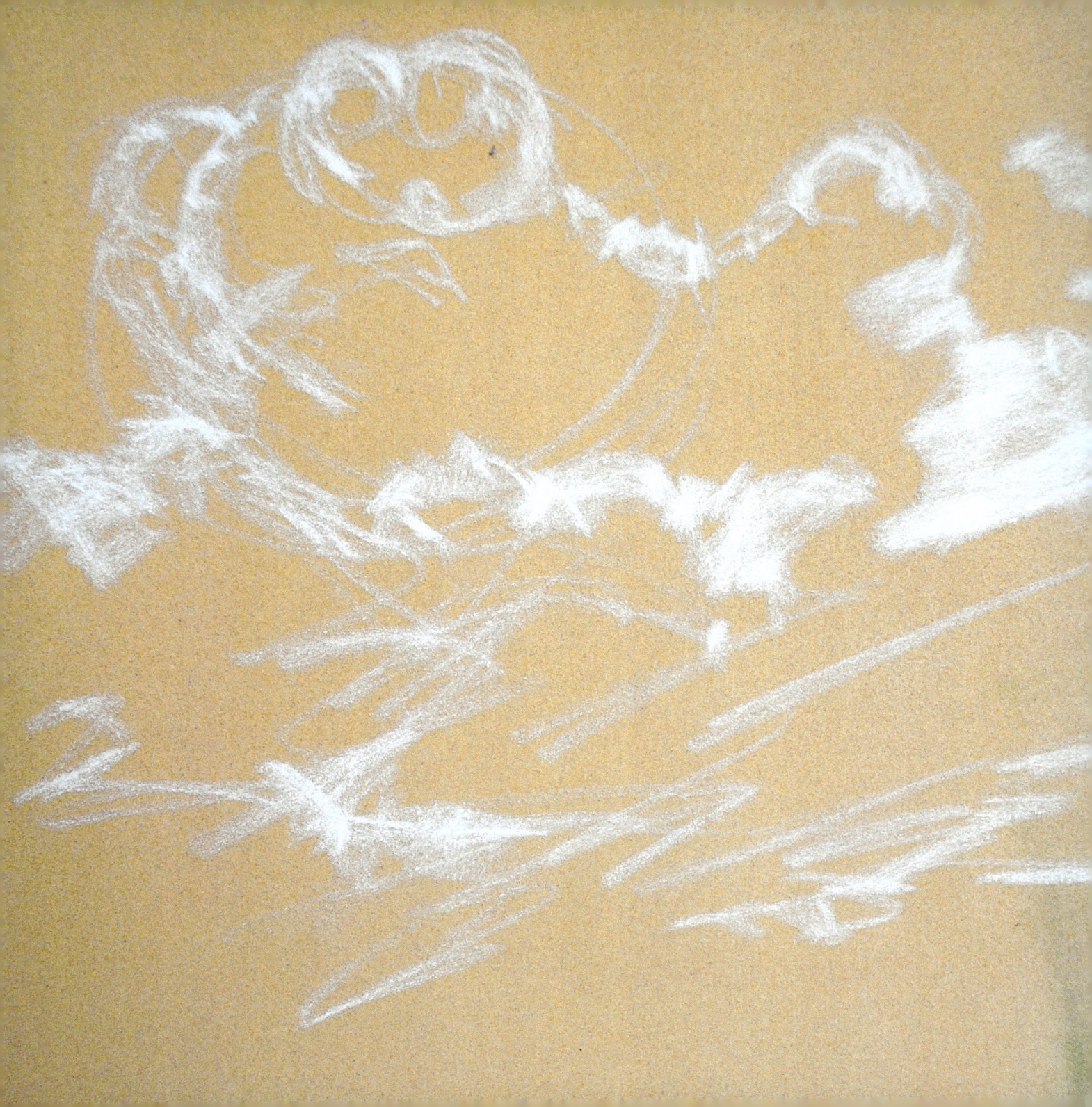

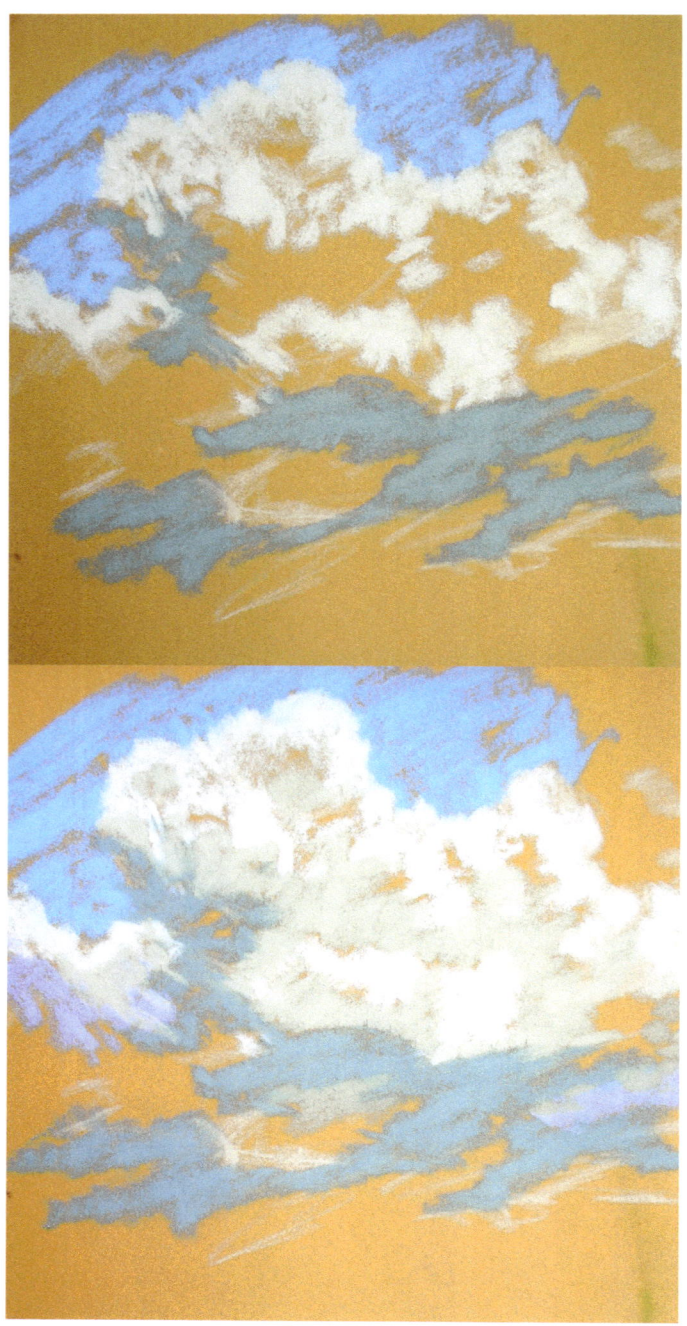

Begin to work on the cloud's interior structure. As clouds become heavier with water moisture, they do not reflect light as well at the top. Refer to your knowledge of how light reflects on a sphere and combine this knowledge along with what you are seeing. Compositions are part seeing, part choosing, and part previous knowledge. This can lead to a painting that looks very realistic or abstracted, whichever is your choice.

Work all over the study, redefining the cloud edges with the sky color. This mid-value blue will ultimately be the cloud's wispy edges and are not as dense as the cloud. Try not to generalize. We all think we know what a cloud looks like, but to sit and study the cloud is a tranquil experience.

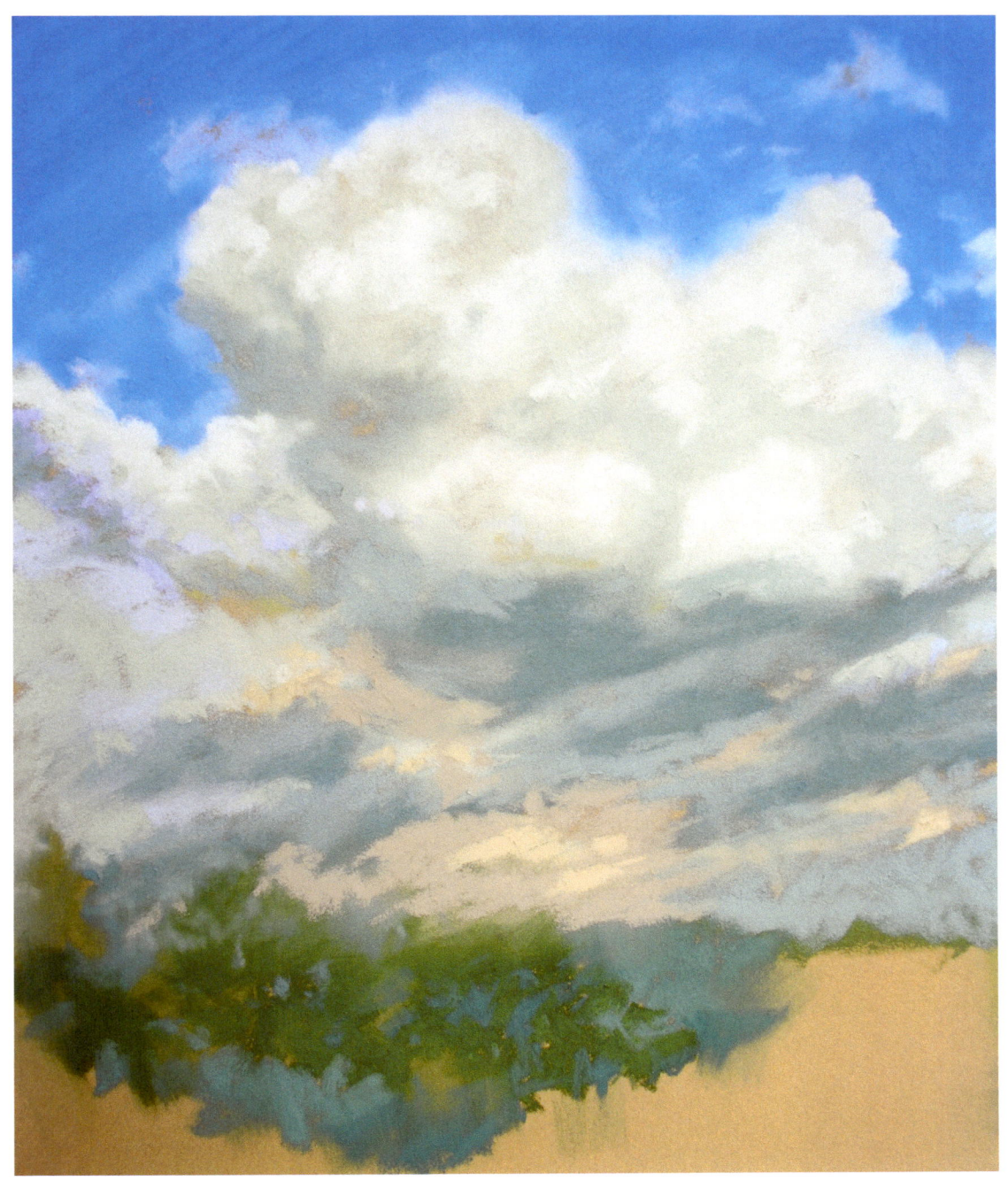

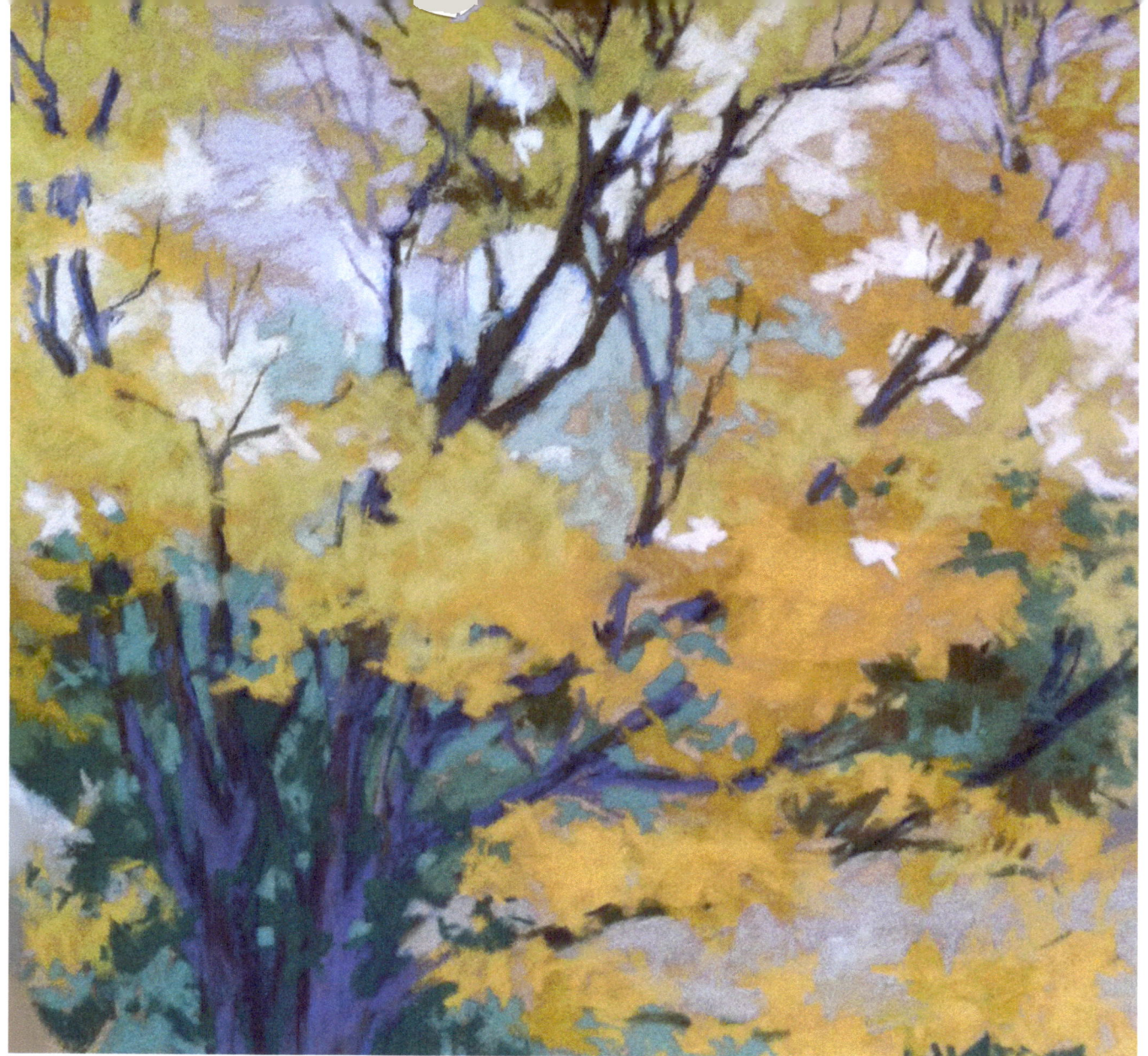

Maple Tree, Pastel, 12 in. x 12 in.
by Alexia Scott, November 2012

Painted from my front door in Falls Church, VA.

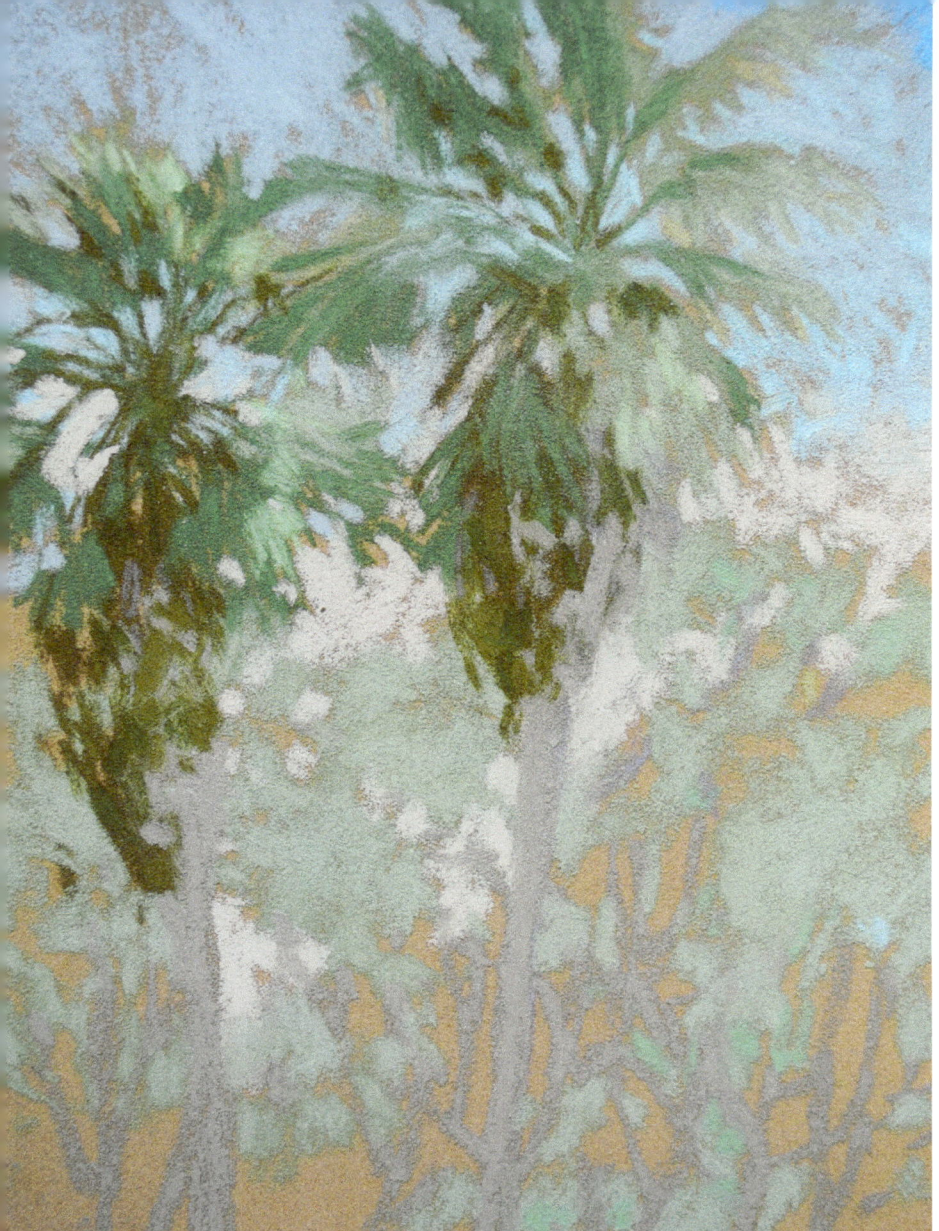

Stuck Inside

Windows provide an "almost as good as" plein air experience. You will miss the sounds of nature but the psychological benefits will be there to recharge your mind. Working from photographs will not have the same effect. Once you paint outside, even with all its challenges, you will find it preferable than working from a photograph. The photograph has no ability to heal your mind from stress. Paint whatever you can see out of any window and make a picture out of it. This is a challenging test and opportunity to review what we have studied and see what you can create within these limiting conditions.

Palm trees study, Pastel, 8 in. x 10 in.
by Alexia Scott, January 2013

Too cold in the morning, this study was done from a hotel window in Carlsbad, CA.

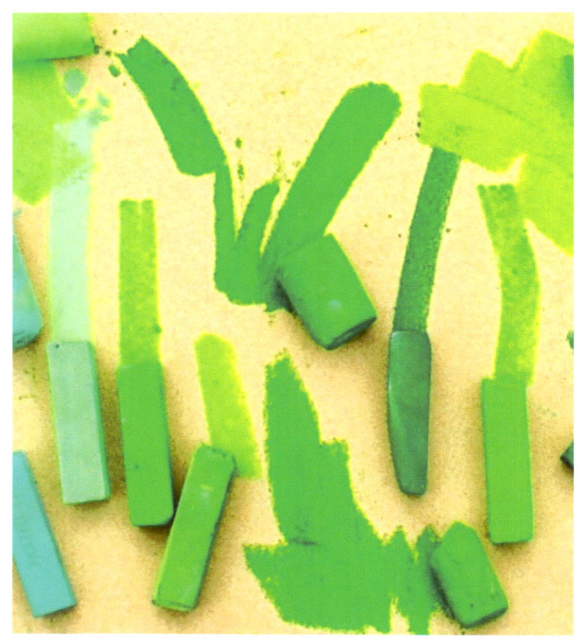

Make Your Mark

Handwriting, which is a lost art in itself, is distinctive from one person to the next. As we grow into adulthood and the Palmer Method of writing is a memory, our strokes take on their own individually unique personalities. Drawing is also unique to the artist making the marks. In a class of 20 art students, I would do a demonstration drawing. We all looked at the same model, but as I walked around the room, I saw 20 very different renderings of the same subject. Fine art is one discipline where copying another artist's work is considered an intelligent strategy for learning, partly because the new work exhibits a little of you.

Pastel painting is both drawing and painting simultaneously. It is the artists' handwriting in a way that does not show up in other forms of two-dimensional work. Again, we are reminded of early man and his/her drawings on cave walls. These drawings are distinctive; and the anthropologist who studied the drawings finds that he/she can identify individual artists. In art history, the drawings produced by an artist are studied for insight into the person that is the artist, much the same as personal letters. There is an intimacy in pastel plein air painting, a new connection between the artist and nature—exploring the landscape, choosing colors, representing a feeling of the time, as well as taking in the view.

Each new day brings new clouds and new light. Flowers bloom and bugs wait to be immortalized in your work.

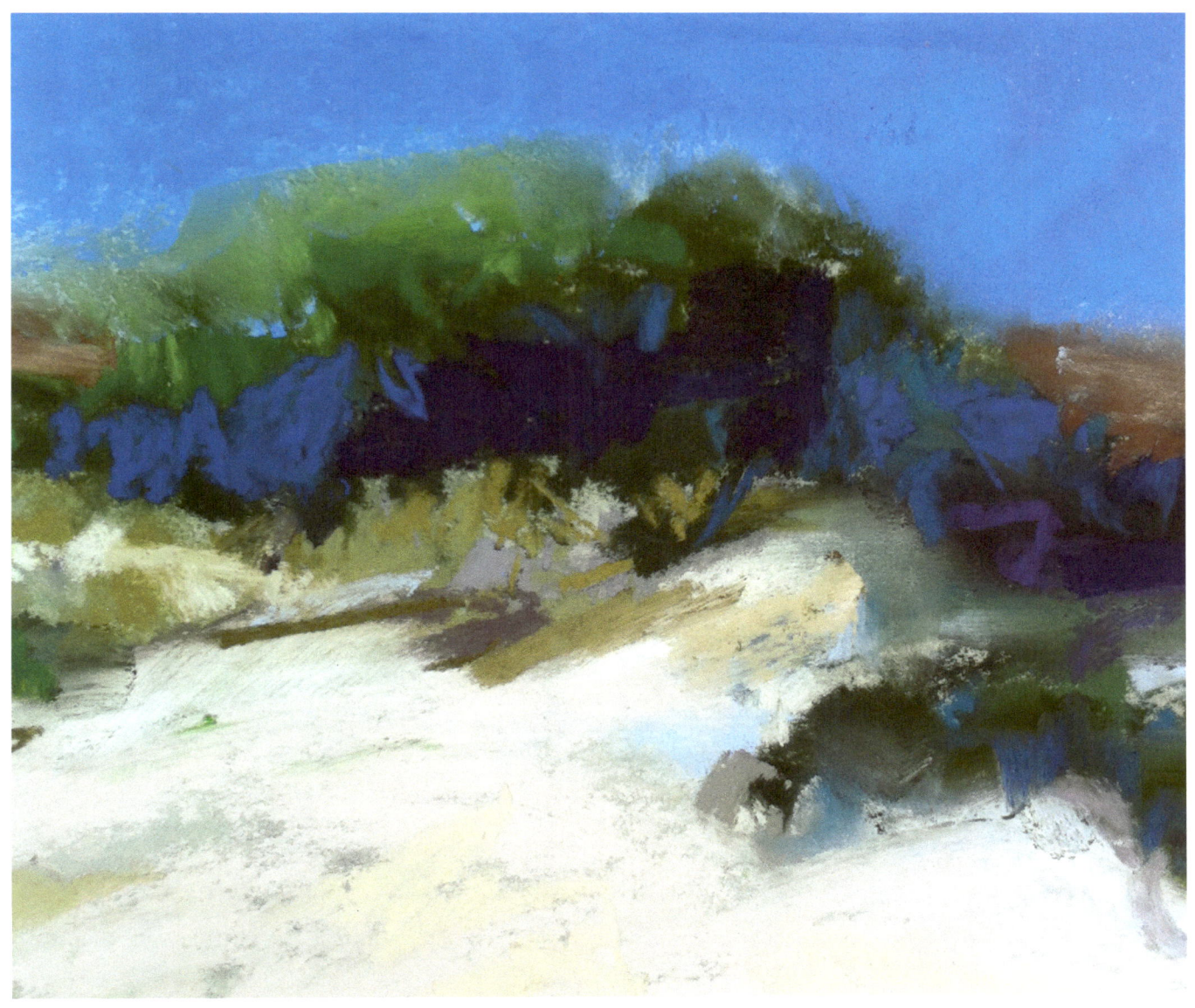

Beach study, Pastel, 5 in. x 5 in.
by Alexia Scott, October 2010

This small pastel from Cape Ann, MA is enlarged to help you see the pastel marks.

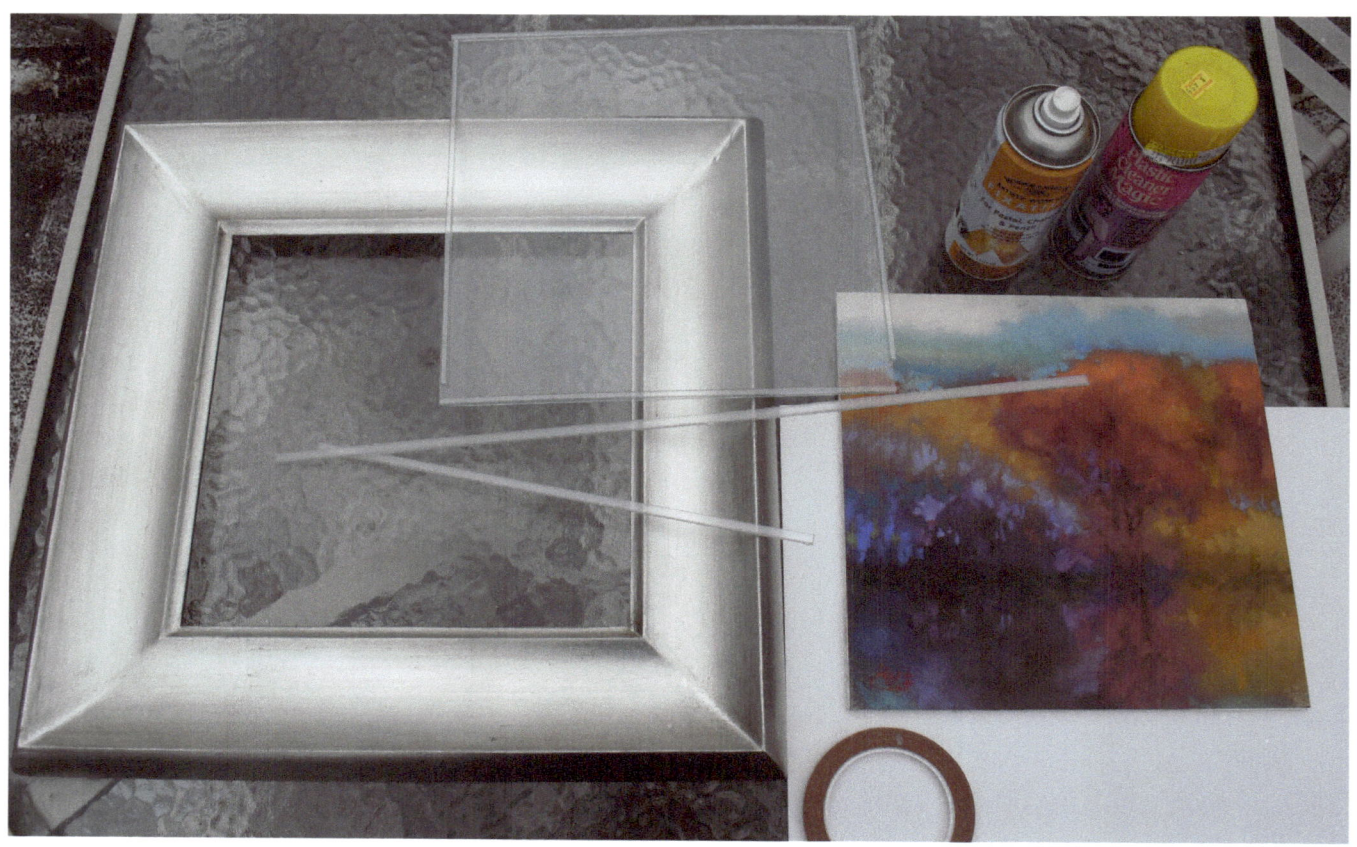

Framing Your Work

Framing a pastel painting is a little different than other paintings. I find it best to give the pastel a little space either through spacers (seen above as plexi sticks) or a mat with pieces of foam core board attached to the mat for spacing. The question as to whether to spray fixative on your pastel is an individual decision.

The Framing Supplies Frame with a three-quarter inch to one inch rabbet depth (distance from the frame lip to the back of the frame). This will give you enough space for the glass, mat, spacing foam core, pastel painting, and protective foam core backing. Find a list of resources and suppliers at www.alexiascottstudio.com.

For your new work, I would suggest picking up ready-made frames that come with all of the contents listed previously. If you want the work to be completely archival, it is best to take it to a framing shop. Pastels are actually very sturdy while under glass. I have pastels drawn by my great-great-grandmother from the 1840's that still look fine. The pure pigments do not fade and the papers are all well-made. Before I frame my work, I decide whether I will spray the painting with fixative. Fixative is a synthetic resin suspended in an alcohol solution. You can spray it on your work to keep the pastel dust from being disturbed. It will often darken your work even after it dries. It is not necessary to spray your work if you are framing it with a space between the glass and the painting. I generally use fixative to set an early under painting and continue drawing, but I rarely spray the painting at the very end.

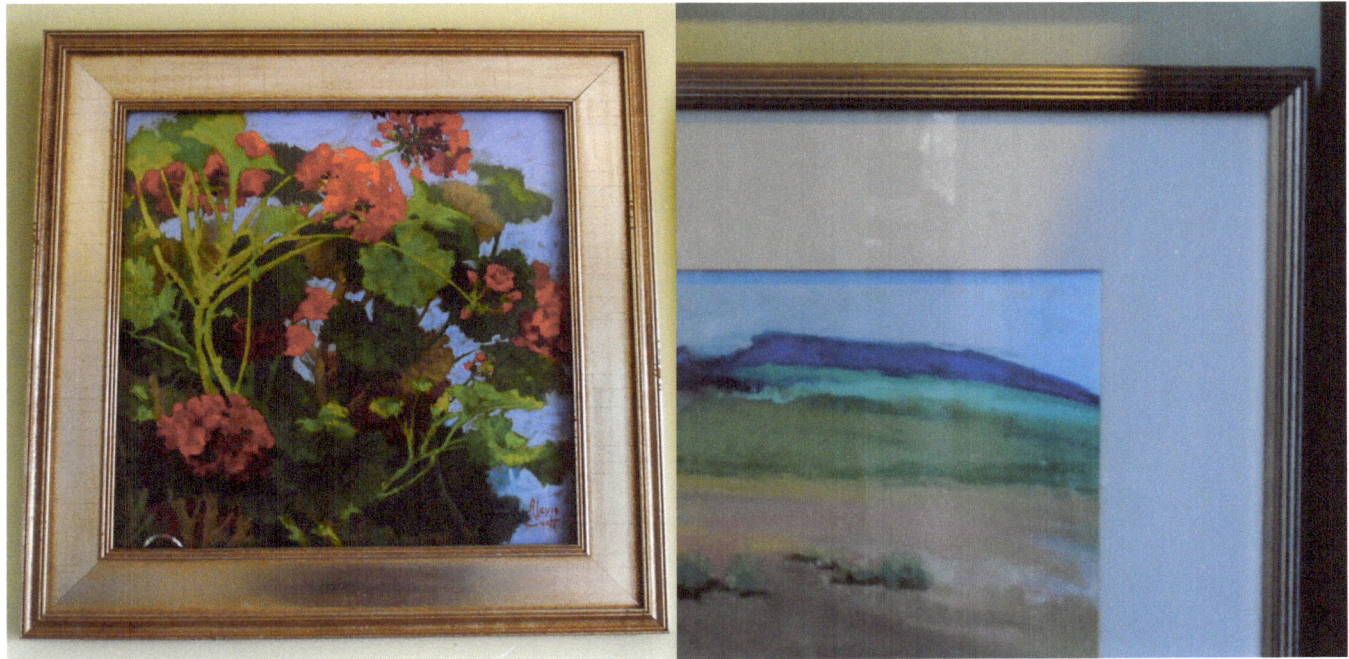

Left Image: Without a mat, add spacers. **Right Image:** With a mat, create a space between the mat and pastel.

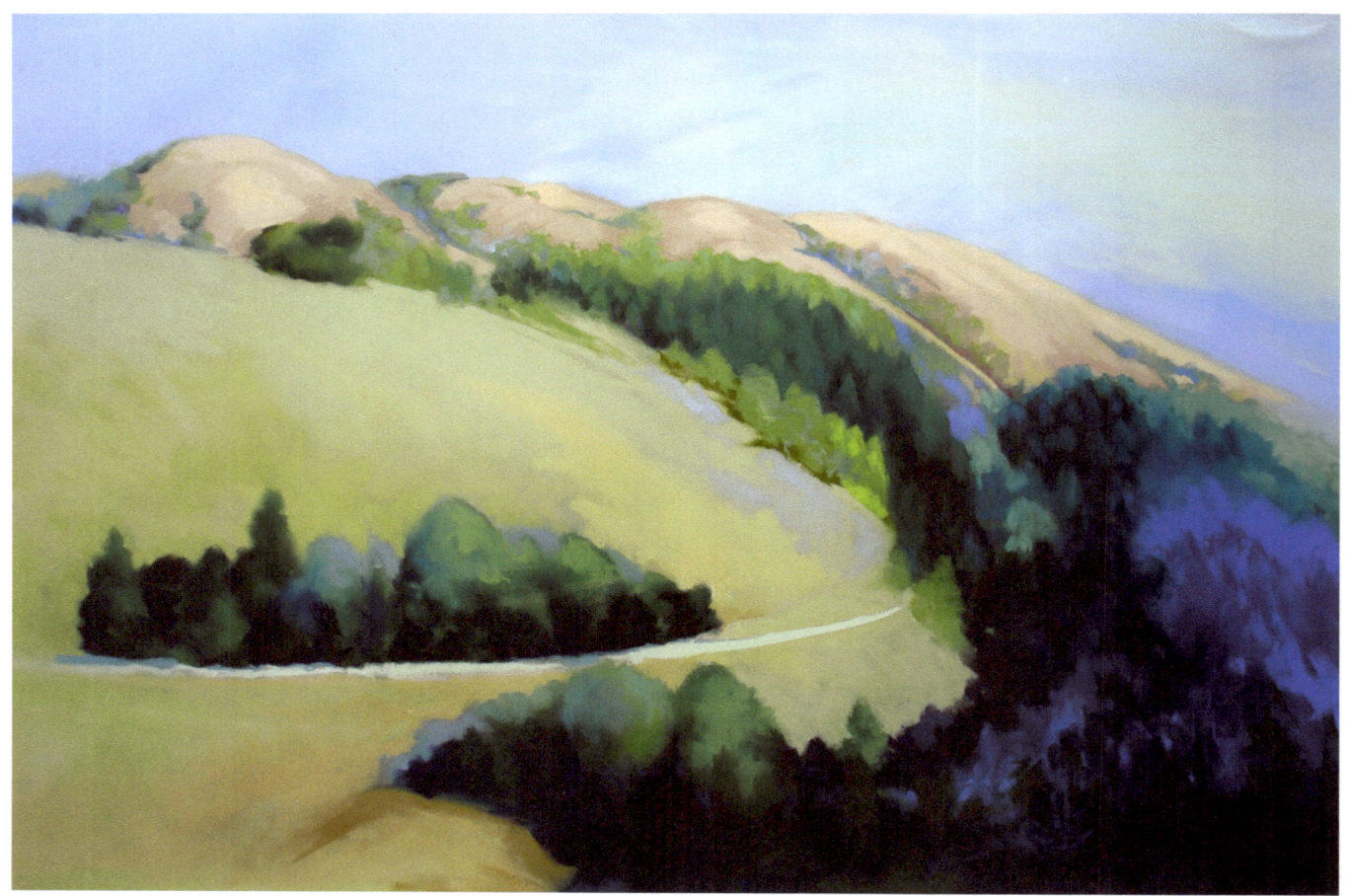

About the Author

Alexia Scott is an American landscape painter. She resides in Northern Virginia but paints both oil and pastel paintings all over the United States. Alexia received her Masters of Fine Arts degree in painting from The George Washington University (GWU). It was at GWU that she had the opportunity to study with artists William Woodward, Helen Frankenthaler, and Wolf Khan. During a visit from Wolf Khan in 1993, her pastels took on renewed importance. Pastel painting emerged from the pastel drawing she had done most of her life.

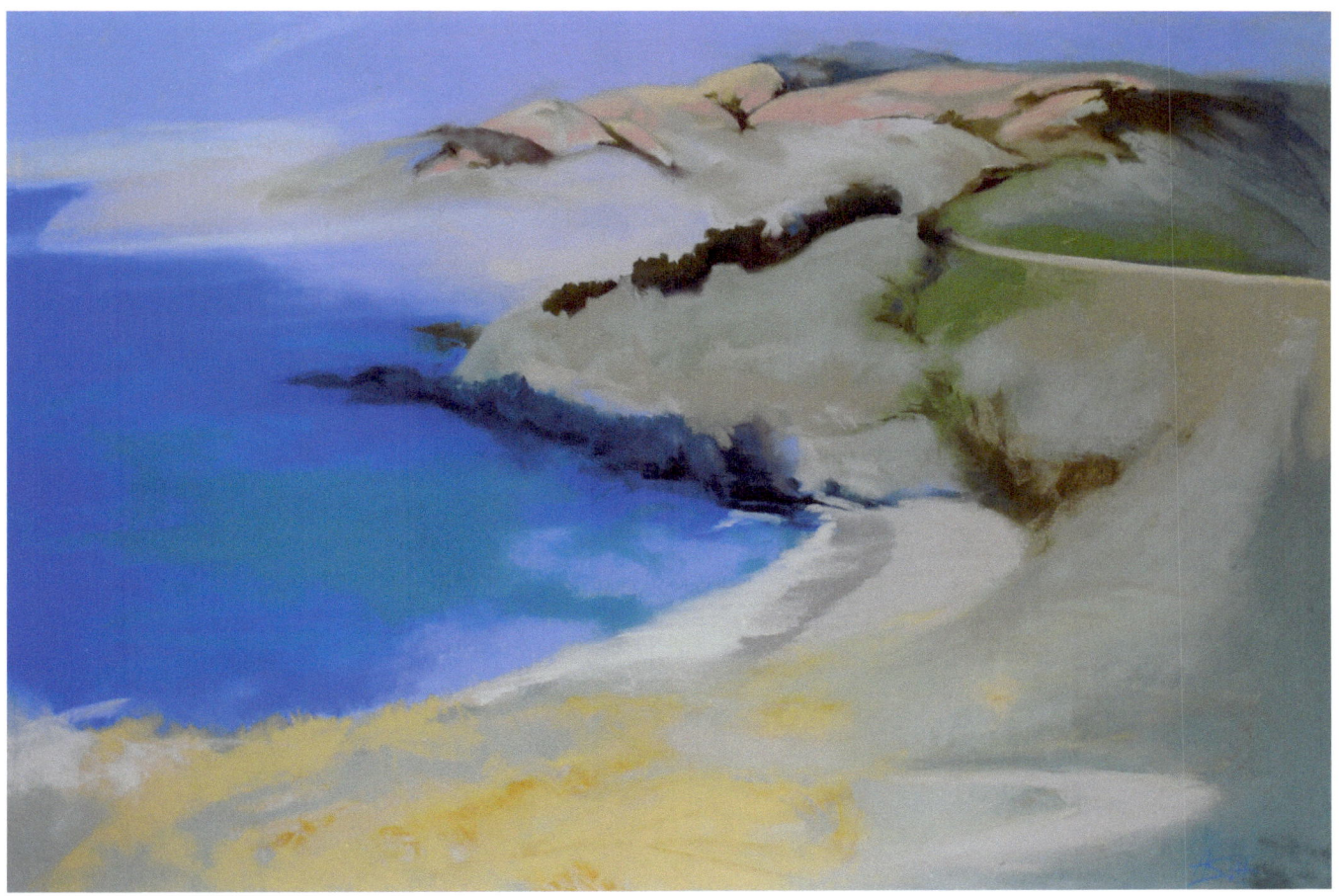

Alexia taught color drawing and color design at Marymount University and fundamental drawing and color drawing at Georgetown University. She exhibits in galleries around the Washington, D.C., area and her work is in private collections, as well as the Smithsonian Zoological Park. She especially enjoys her time spent in nature with her pastels while visiting our National Parks. To quote Ken Burns: "The parks allowed us to arrest—if only for a few hours—the momentum and distractions of our lives, and give us, out in nature, a chance to connect to our best selves."

Left Image: *Behind Nepenthe Big Sur*, Pastel on Wallis white sanded paper, by Alexia Scott
This page: *Big Sur California*, Pastel on Wallis white sanded paper, by Alexia Scott

You can view more of Alexia's work at **www.alexiascottstudio.com**

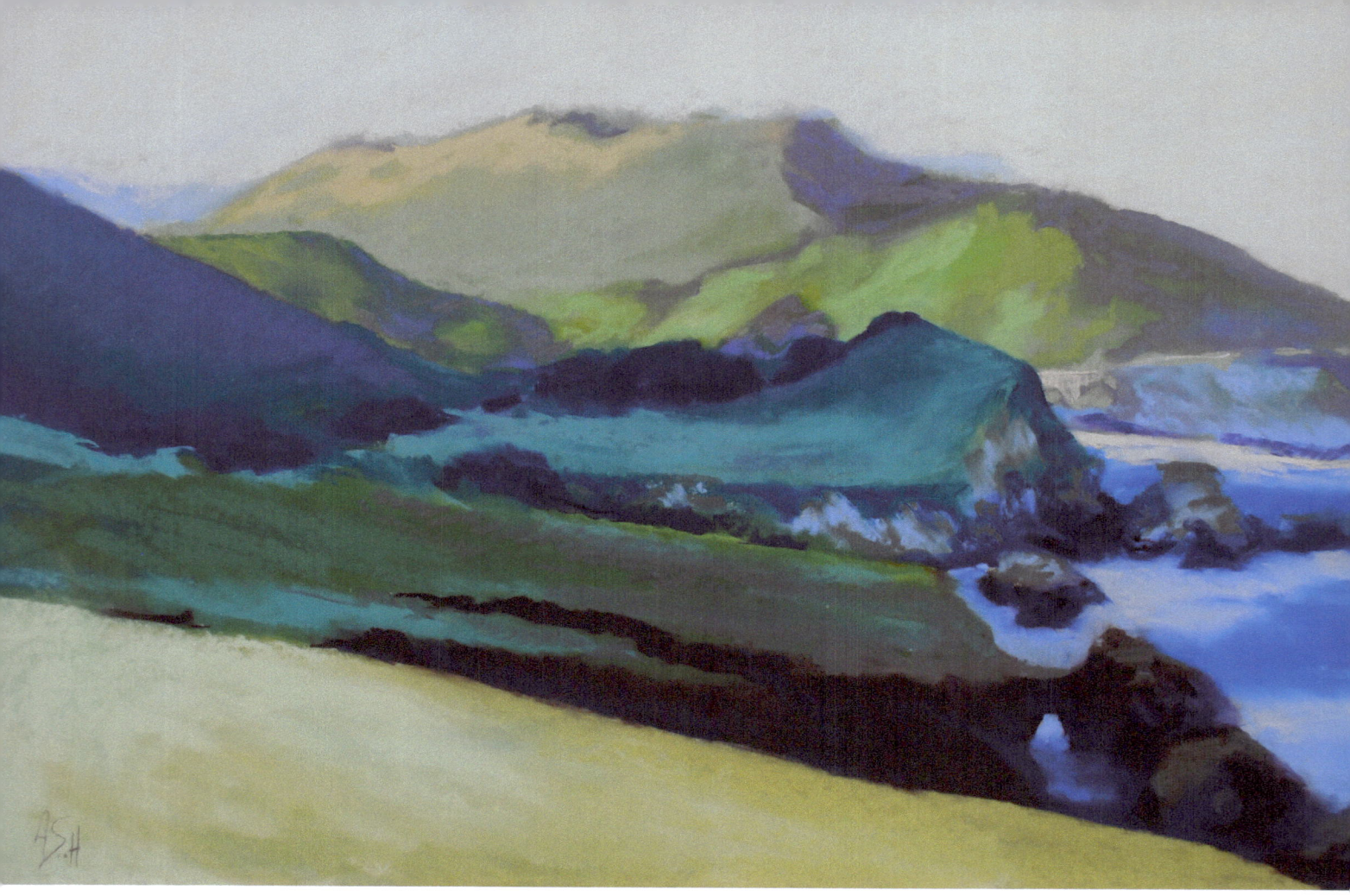

A special thanks to my mother, Priscilla Smith Scheffler, who painted up and down the Pacific Coast during World War II while my dad, who was in the U.S. Navy, was stationed in San Diego, CA, and Bremerton, WA. I not only grew up with a family who loved art, but loved the scenic beauty of America. By the age of 18, I had visited 48 states by automobile and painted with my mother on Cape Cod, MA.

www.ingramcontent.com/pod-product-compliance
Lightning Source LLC
Chambersburg PA
CBHW041459280526
45792CB00004B/1059